Mayo Clinic on *Vision and Eye Health*

Helmut Buettner, M.D.

Editor in Chief

Mayo Clinic
Rochester, Minnesota

Mayo Clinic on Vision and Eye Health provides reliable, practical information on eye care and safety, the signs and symptoms of serious eye disorders, and the diagnosis and treatment of these disorders. Much of this information comes directly from the experience of ophthalmologists, optometrists and other health care professionals at Mayo Clinic. This book supplements the advice of your physician, whom you should consult for individual problems you may be having with your vision. *Mayo Clinic on Vision and Eye Health* does not endorse any company or product. MAYO, MAYO CLINIC, MAYO CLINIC HEALTH INFORMATION and the Mayo triple-shield logo are marks of Mayo Foundation for Medical Education and Research.

Published by Mayo Clinic Health Information, Rochester, Minn. Distributed to the book trade by Kensington Publishing Corporation, New York, N.Y.

Photo credits: Cover photos and the photos on pages 1, 51, 56, 57, 63, 81, 89, 99, 107 and 114 are from PhotoDisc®.

Library of Congress Catalog Card Number: 2001 135099

ISBN 1-893005-20-8

Printed in the United States of America

First Edition

1 2 3 4 5 6 7 8 9 10

About vision

With proper care your vision can function splendidly into old age. But the delicate structures of your eye can change as you get older, making it harder to see as well as you once did. Aging also puts you at increased risk of serious eye disorders, especially after you're in your 60s or older. Disorders such as glaucoma, cataracts and macular degeneration are virtually undetectable in their early stages without the help of an eye specialist. And if untreated they can seriously impair your vision and may permanently rob you of sight.

The good news is that most eye diseases are treatable if they're diagnosed early. Living with impaired vision is made easier with the assistance of technology and special training. The keys are regular eye examinations and common-sense precautions in your day-to-day life. This book, based on the expertise of Mayo Clinic doctors, can help you with decisions you need to make to keep your eyes healthy and enjoy good vision.

About Mayo Clinic

Mayo Clinic evolved from the frontier practice of Dr. William Worrall Mayo and the partnership of his two sons, William J. and Charles H. Mayo, in the early 1900s. Pressed by the demands of their busy practice in Rochester, Minn., the Mayo brothers invited other physicians to join them, pioneering the private group practice of medicine. Today, with more than 2,000 physicians and scientists at its three major locations in Rochester, Minn., Jacksonville, Fla., and Scottsdale, Ariz., Mayo Clinic is dedicated to providing comprehensive diagnoses, accurate answers, and effective treatments.

With this depth of medical knowledge, experience and expertise, Mayo Clinic occupies an unparalleled position as a health information resource. Since 1983 Mayo Clinic has published reliable health information for millions of consumers through award-winning newsletters, books and online services. Revenue from the publishing activities supports Mayo Clinic programs, including medical education and research.

Editorial staff

Editor in Chief
Helmut Buettner, M.D.

Managing Editor
Kevin Kaufman

Copy Editor
Mary Duerson

Proofreaders
Miranda Attlesey
Donna Hanson
Karen Kulzer

Editorial Researchers
Anthony Cook
Deirdre Herman
Michelle Hewlett

Contributing Writers
Lee Engfer
Rebecca Gonzalez-Campoy
Stephen Miller

Creative Director
Daniel Brevick

Layout and Production Artist
Stewart J. Koski
Paul Krause

Illustrators and Photographers
Thomas Link
Richard Madsen
Jay Rostvold
Christopher Srnka

Indexer
Larry Harrison

Contributing editors and reviewers

Keith Baratz, M.D.
Tracy M. Berg, R.Ph.
Jay Erie, M.D.

David Herman, M.D.
Dennis Siemsen, O.D.,
M.H.P.E.

Preface

A primary focus of this book is the impact of aging on our eyes. Some of us from childhood on have had difficulties focusing on objects close up or far away, and that may have been the extent of our vision problems for many years. On reaching our 40s or 50s, this may no longer hold true. The natural process of aging is not always kind to our eyes. Years of wear and tear can cloud the lens or make it less elastic. Suddenly we find we can no longer read fine print without holding the paper at arm's length. On reaching our 60s, we face an increased risk of eye disorders such as glaucoma, macular degeneration and cataracts.

Nevertheless, good eye care and common-sense precautions may allow your eyes to function properly and well serve your needs into old age. You can take many simple measures in your everyday life to keep your eyes healthy. We also have the means — such as eyeglasses, contact lenses and now even surgery — to correct many flaws of imperfect vision. Early treatment can halt or delay the progress of serious eye disorders. Surgeons can repair a detached retina or implant an artificial lens.

In the pages that follow, you'll learn about the amazing complexity and sophistication of your eyes. You'll be guided through the steps of an eye exam and the choices that may be available to you if you have vision problems. You'll find detailed and easy-to-understand explanations of many eye disorders — some common, some rare. This knowledge can help you in preparing for various treatment options.

We believe that the more you know about your eyes, the longer you'll benefit from and enjoy healthy vision. And the best way to preserve vision is by recognizing the onset of eye problems. Early action minimizes eye damage and greatly reduces the extent and complexity of treatment. Along with the advice of your eye doctor, this book can help you live well and experience the richness and pleasure of sight.

Helmut Buettner, M.D.
Editor in Chief

Contents

Part 1

How you see

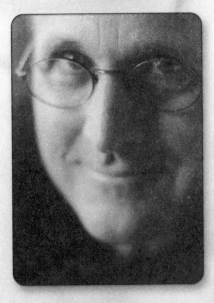

Chapter 1

A look inside

Your eyes are such a small part of your body. Each eyeball is about an inch in diameter, just a little smaller than the ball used for table tennis. Yet your eyes play such a big role in your life. With them you experience the shape, the color and the motion of your surroundings. They alert you to danger or the unexpected. You rely on them to explore or learn. Of your five senses — sight, hearing, touch, smell and taste — sight is the sense you've likely come to trust most in your everyday activities. With the help of your eyes, you read books, write notes, balance your checkbook, drive your car, do your work, fix your meals and care for your loved ones. On an emotional level, your vision helps to define your self-image and your personal interactions with others. Author Henry David Thoreau expressed it succinctly, "We are as much as we see." Given how much you depend on your eyes, it's no wonder you want to keep them as healthy as you possibly can.

Your eyes at work

People often compare eyes to a camera, and there are similarities. Like a camera each eye lets light enter into the interior through a small opening. An adjustable lens focuses the light onto a layer of light-sensitive cells at the back of the eyeball, comparable to the light-sensitive film in the camera.

This comparison, however, doesn't do your eyes justice. They are far more complex and sophisticated than a camera or any other technology. For one thing it's a pair of eyeballs we're talking about, which move and function together in perfect synchronization. The eyeball covering is super flexible, resilient and lightweight. Each eyeball autoregulates many rapid adjustments for brightness, focus and internal pressure. Light striking the back of each eyeball induces chemical reactions that generate electric impulses. These impulses trigger two-way communication between the eyes and a command center in the brain. By way of this communication, your eyeballs provide binocular vision and follow rapid movement. All of these features give you vivid, colorful, three-dimensional motion pictures faster than you can blink an eye, literally.

Here's a description of the various, intricate parts of the eye and how they work together. Each part plays an essential role in the healthy functioning of the eye. And each part can be responsible for particular eye problems.

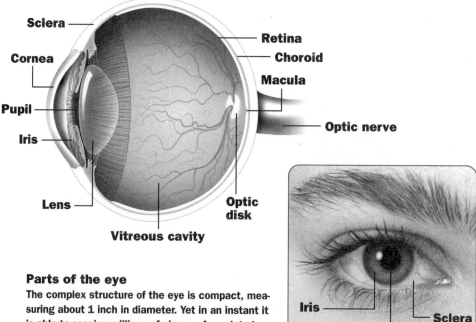

Parts of the eye

The complex structure of the eye is compact, measuring about 1 inch in diameter. Yet in an instant it is able to receive millions of pieces of unrelated information about the outside world.

Orbit

Your eyes are cradled in the orbits, which are sockets formed by a protective structure of heavy bone. This structure includes the cheekbone, forehead bone, temple bone and bridge of your nose. Unlike other bones in your body, these eye protectors usually don't weaken and thin with age. Small pillows of fat cushion the eyeball within the orbit.

Upper and lower eyelids protect the front of your eyeball by blocking dirt and bright light that can damage your eyes. The eyelids also lubricate your eyeball with each blink, which happens every few seconds. Blinking washes away dust, pollen and other foreign bodies. The lubricant, familiar to us as tears, comes from glands above each eye. When something irritates your eye, such as chemical vapor from the onion you're peeling, the tear glands open their faucets. If tearing is slight, the fluid will drain through tiny ducts within each eyelid and into your nose, taking the irritants with it. But the drainage system can't handle fully opened faucets. That's when tears overflow and run down your cheeks, such as when you're crying.

Sclera

When you look in the mirror and see the white of your eye, you're looking at the sclera — the tough, white, leathery coating that forms the circular eyeball shape and protects the delicate internal structures of the eye. The sclera has an opening at the front that allows light inside the eyeball.

A thin, moist, clear membrane called the conjunctiva covers the exposed front portion of the sclera. This tissue layer folds forward to also line the inside of your eyelids. The conjunctiva helps lubricate your eye.

Cornea

At the front of your eye, covering the opening in the sclera like a protective window, is a domed layer of clear tissue called the cornea. It juts out from the eyeball as a tiny bulge. The convex surface of the cornea bends the light entering your eye. This action is the initial, large-scale focusing of the object you're looking at, leaving the lens to fine-tune and sharpen the focus of the image.

The cornea, which is made up of several layers of tissue, also protects your eye. It's packed with sensitive nerve endings. When even a tiny speck of dust hits the cornea, you get the message instantly. If tears can't wash away the foreign material, the continuing pain prods you to locate and remove it.

Pupil

That dark spot in the center of your eye is a hole — somewhat like the dark opening of a cave. It's through this hole, which is covered by your cornea, that light passes into your eye (see figure 1a in the color section).

Iris

Surrounding your pupil is the iris, the colored part of your eye. Its color comes from a pigment called melanin in your iris tissue. The more pigment, the darker the color. Brown eyes have a lot of pigment. Blue or green eyes have less pigment. As you get older, the color may change as your iris loses some of this pigment.

But the iris adds more than color to your eye. The iris contains a ring of muscle fibers that can expand or contract the size of the

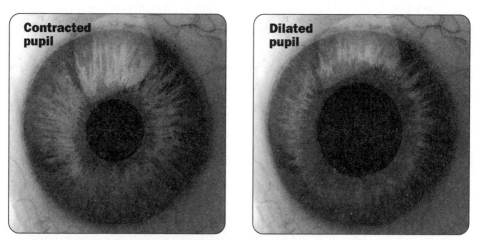

Adjustments of the iris to light conditions
The iris adjusts the size of the pupil according to light conditions. In normal light the average pupil is open a little more than a tenth of an inch, about half the size of a pencil eraser. But its diameter can range from about six one-hundredths of an inch in bright light to about a third of an inch in low light.

pupil, and thereby control the amount of light that gets inside the eyeball. It's a bit like adjusting blinds to control the amount of sunlight coming through a window. When the light is bright, the iris reacts quickly to reduce the size of the pupil. When the light is dim, the iris enlarges the size of the pupil.

The muscles of your iris can react to more than light. Your emotions affect the size of your pupils. Anger can make them smaller. Excitement and pleasure can open them wider. Certain drugs can open (dilate) the pupils. Eye doctors use dilating drugs to get a better look inside your eyes during an examination.

The space between your cornea and iris is called the anterior chamber. It's filled with a clear fluid called aqueous humor, which nourishes the cornea and the lens, washes away waste products, and plays an important role in maintaining pressure in the eye.

Lens

Behind the iris and pupil is the lens, a clear, elliptical structure about the size and shape of an M&M's candy. A circular muscle surrounds the lens. As the muscle relaxes or contracts, the lens curvature changes to sharpen the focus of whatever you're looking at.

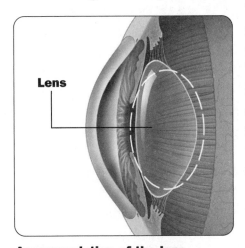

When an object is nearby, the muscle contracts and the lens thickens by its own elasticity. When an object is far away, the muscle relaxes and the lens stretches thin. These adjustments, known as accommodation, allow the lens to change its focusing power and sharpen the definition of the objects you're looking at. This variable focusing power fine-tunes the fixed focusing power of your cornea. As you get older, your lens can lose its elasticity, and you may have difficulty focusing on objects close by.

Accommodation of the lens
Changes in the shape of the lens accommodate distance vision (solid line) and close-up vision (dashed line). The thicker the lens, the more the light is refracted and the more close up the eye can see.

20/20 vision

It's great when an eye doctor says you have 20/20 vision. But that doesn't mean you have perfect vision. It simply means that you can see objects clearly from 20 feet away that an average of normal-sighted people can see clearly from 20 feet away. In other words it's a measure of your visual acuity — how sharply or clearly you can see something at a distance.

If you're nearsighted and have 20/50 vision, that means distant objects are fuzzy. In fact they're so fuzzy that what you see from 20 feet away is what people with normal vision generally can see from 50 feet away. Some people have sharper vision than 20/20. Some have 20/15 vision, or even 20/10.

There is no such thing as perfect vision. That's because many factors other than visual acuity affect your ability to see well. Even if you can see what you should from 20 feet away, your doctor will want to check your depth perception, color vision, peripheral vision and ability to focus on close objects. Many of these indicators are tested in a routine eye examination.

Vitreous cavity

The vitreous cavity extends from the back of the lens to the retina at the back of the eyeball. It is filled with a clear, gelatinous substance called the vitreous humor or, simply, the vitreous. Together with the aqueous humor in the anterior chamber, the vitreous helps maintain the pressure and shape of the eyeball.

In order for light to pass through it, the vitreous is clear. You may occasionally notice what look like tiny bits of string or lint darting through your vision. These are called floaters, tiny bits of material forming in the vitreous. A sudden onset of or increase in floaters, especially when associated with flashing lights or hazy vision, can be a sign of potentially serious eye problems.

Retina

On the inside back wall of the eyeball is a thin layer of tissue called the retina (see figure 1b in the color section). This term comes from a Latin word meaning "net." It's an apt name because your retina consists of millions of light-sensitive cells and nerve cells that capture the images focused onto them by your cornea and lens.

The light-sensitive cells (sometimes called photoreceptors) are either rods or cones. There are about 20 rod cells for every cone cell. Rod cells allow you to see in very dim light or off to the side while looking ahead (peripheral, or side, vision), but they can't distinguish colors. Cone cells distinguish color exquisitely but require more light to function. This is why it can be hard to see color in the evening or in dim light. (Hence the saying, "At night all cats are gray.") Cone cells are concentrated in the center of your retina and allow you to see sharp detail when you're looking straight ahead at a well-lit object.

Light striking the rods and cones triggers a chemical reaction. This in turn generates electrical impulses that are relayed through the optic nerve to the visual cortex, the seeing portion of your brain. The image that your retina receives is upside-down. It's also reversed, similar to how you see a reversed image of yourself when you look in a mirror. These effects are caused by the convex shape of both the cornea and the lens. Your brain reinterprets this information, allowing you to see the images in their correct orientation. The brain must also merge the image from both eyes to produce a clear picture.

The outer part of your retina is nourished mainly by the choroid, a layer of arteries and veins sandwiched between the retina and the sclera. The inner part of the retina receives its nutrition from retinal blood vessels.

Macula and fovea

At the center of your retina is the macula, which is densely packed with cone cells. This dark reddish patch is the part of your retina that provides your central, or straight-ahead, vision and allows you to see fine detail. It's used for reading and other close-up work. Within the macula is a small depression called the fovea, which contains only cone cells and provides your sharpest vision.

Outside the macula your retina contains primarily rod cells, which can't process images as sharply as the cone cells in the macula but are responsible for peripheral and night vision.

Optic nerve

The visual information gathered by your retina is carried to the visual cortex of your brain by a bundle of over 1 million nerve fibers. This communication cable between your eyes and your brain is called the optic nerve. The brain instantly decodes the visual impulses, coordinating signals from both eyes to produce a three-dimensional image.

A yellowish circle visible on the retina is where the optic nerve forms at the back of the eye. This location is called the optic disk.

Muscles of the eyeball

Each eyeball has six muscles attached to the sclera, allowing you to move both eyes and track an object without necessarily turning your head. These eye muscles, working individually or together, allow you to shift your visual field left, right, up, down and diagonally. Your brain coordinates these eye movements, so the eyes move in unison when tracking an object.

Common vision problems

The intricate process of vision, which has so many complex parts and interactions, can sometimes go wrong. The four most common vision problems — nearsightedness, farsightedness, astigmatism and presbyopia — are usually caused by focusing problems of the cornea or the lens or by an abnormal shape of the eye. Most problems with focusing can be corrected with eyeglasses, contact lenses or surgery that adjusts the curvature of your cornea.

You see an object clearly when it is properly focused. That means your cornea and lens have adjusted the point of focus so that an image falls sharply defined onto your retina. If the focusing powers of your cornea and lens aren't coordinated with the length or the shape of your eye, however, the image you see is blurred.

Nearsightedness

If you're nearsighted — a condition called myopia (mi-O-pe-uh) — you can see objects that are near to you clearly, but objects farther away are blurry. You're nearsighted if your eyeball is elongated from front to back rather than round. This causes the object you're looking at to be sharply focused in front of the retina instead of on the retina. Even with a round eye you can be nearsighted if your cornea or lens is too steeply curved.

Nearsightedness is a common problem, affecting nearly 3 out of 10 people. Many people first notice the condition during childhood when, for example, they have trouble making out what the teacher writes on the board at school. It affects boys and girls equally and tends to run in families. The problem can progress quickly during these early years, sometimes requiring new corrective lenses more than once a year. Vision tends to stabilize during the young adult years, so during your 20s and 30s you may not need a change in your lenses.

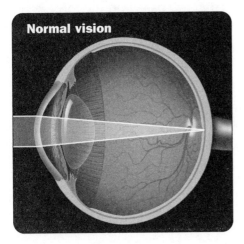

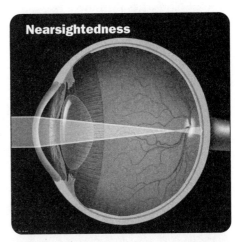

Common vision problems

With normal vision the image is sharply focused onto your retina. With nearsightedness the point of focus is in front of your retina, making distant objects appear blurry. With farsightedness the point of focus falls behind your retina, making close-up objects appear blurry.

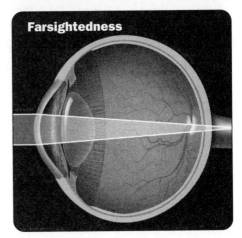

Colorblindness

Most people who have what's called colorblindness aren't really colorblind. That would mean they see only black and white. Actually, their problem is that it's hard to tell the difference between certain shades of color. Most people with colorblindness can't tell the difference between red and green. Others can't tell the difference between shades of blue and yellow.

The problem is usually inherited, though eye diseases and some medicines also can cause it. About 8 percent of men and 1 percent of women are born having trouble with their color discrimination. Some people are simply unaware of their color vision problems.

The problem arises from color pigment deficiencies in the cone cells in your retina. These pigments allow you to distinguish between many hues of colors that are based on the three primary colors: red, blue and green. If you're missing one or more color pigments, you may see only two of the primary colors. Confusing the red light and the green light of a traffic signal is a well-known problem associated with colorblindness. People with colorblindness may also be unable to distinguish ripening fruit and vegetables in a garden, for example, a tomato changing color from green to red.

Doctors can diagnose color vision deficiencies and determine their severity. There's no cure for the inherited forms of colorblindness. However, if a disease causes poor color vision, treatment may slow or reverse the deficiency. Doctors can also suggest ways you can compensate for the problem. Specially tinted eyeglasses may help you distinguish between confusing colors. And you can learn to recognize colors by their brightness and location, such as the positions of the red light and the green light on a traffic signal.

Concave lenses, which are thinner in the middle than at the edges, can correct myopia. You can wear the lenses as glasses or contacts. Another way of correcting this problem — refractive surgery — is growing in popularity. It's a brief procedure that reduces the curvature of your cornea so that the light entering your eye focuses directly on your retina again. Two types of refractive surgery are photorefractive keratectomy and LASIK surgery (see pages 46 to 50).

Farsightedness

When you're farsighted — a condition called hyperopia (hi-pur-O-pe-uh) — you may see objects that are far away clearly but have difficulty focusing on objects close to you.

In most cases people are farsighted because their eyeball is shorter than normal from front to back. The rays of light coming into the eye aren't sharply focused at the time they reach the retina. Instead the point of focus falls behind the retina. This problem can also be caused by either a cornea or a lens that doesn't have a steep enough curvature.

Farsightedness runs in families and is usually present at birth. Most young people don't know they have the condition because their lens is flexible and able to accomodate enough to focus the light sharply on the retina. But constant overworking of the muscles that make your lens assume a more tightly curved shape can leave you with aching or burning eyes, headaches, fatigue or blurred vision after you've done a lot of reading or close-up work. As you grow older your lens becomes less elastic and unable to make the necessary shape adjustment. Most farsighted people need corrective lenses by middle age.

The correction of farsightedness is accomplished with a convex lens, which is thicker in the center than at the edges. This moves the point of focus forward, onto the surface of your retina. Surgery also is an option that's becoming more popular, but the procedure is complicated and therefore is not performed as commonly as the surgery to correct nearsightedness.

Astigmatism

In a normal eye the dome of your cornea is curved evenly and smoothly in all directions. This allows for the round ball that you are looking at, for example, to be focused perfectly on your retina and thus be perceived as a round ball. Some corneas, however,

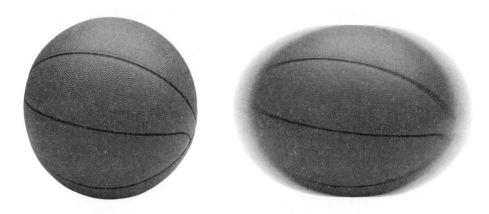

How astigmatism affects vision

Astigmatism is caused by the uneven curvature of your cornea, which is unable to focus the light entering your eye evenly and creates distorted, blurry vision. A round basketball (left) appears oblong (right) because the cornea is curved more sharply up and down than side to side.

aren't evenly and smoothly curved. Instead they are curved more steeply in one direction than in another. A round ball viewed through such a cornea will be seen as oblong. Typically you'll see the distortion in one direction more than in others, either horizontally, vertically or diagonally. This distortion of the image is called astigmatism (uh-STIG-muh-tiz-um).

Astigmatism is in most instances inherited, but sometimes it may develop following an injury or a disease. About half the people who are nearsighted also have some astigmatism. The condition generally doesn't change throughout your life.

You may not notice the distortion caused by minor degrees of astigmatism. More serious astigmatism can be corrected with a cylindrical lens that counteracts the uneven curvature of your cornea. The same lens you use to correct nearsightedness or farsightedness can be made to neutralize your astigmatism as well. Another option is surgery to reshape the curvature of your cornea — it is similar to the surgery used to correct nearsightedness and farsightedness.

Presbyopia

Although the term *presbyopia* (pres-be-O-pe-uh) may be unfamiliar to you, the condition probably isn't. It's a Greek word meaning

Second sight

Some older adults are surprised — and delighted — by what is called second sight. After using reading glasses or bifocals for many years, you suddenly discover that your vision has improved. You no longer need the reading correction.

This happens when the lens of your eye becomes thicker as you age. It produces some nearsightedness, which can correct your presbyopia at the same time. However, not all of the news is good. The vision change is usually a sign that a cataract is forming, which ultimately clouds your vision. So it's a good idea to inform your eye doctor if you notice the development of second sight.

"old sight." About the time you're 40 or older, you may notice that it's harder to read at the distance you are accustomed to. The print seems smaller, and you have to hold papers farther away, sometimes at arm's length, to get them in focus.

If you're already farsighted, you may encounter the problem earlier in life. If you're nearsighted you'll eventually experience presbyopia, although later in life than a normal-sighted person. It's a natural part of aging. When you're young the lens in your eye is very elastic, giving you a wide range of focus. The lens becomes thicker when you're reading, sewing or doing other close-up work. This thickening adjusts the point of focus so that it falls on your retina. As you get older your lens gradually loses its elasticity and ability to change shape. You can no longer properly focus on objects close to you without the help of corrective lenses.

People who are nearsighted may find they can do tasks like reading simply by taking off their distance glasses. But in time many of them likely will need glasses for close-up work as well. Another correction for nearsighted people is to wear a different strength of contact lens on each eye. Your dominant eye — usually the one you'll use for aiming or picture taking — gets the correction for seeing at a distance, and the other eye gets the correction for reading and seeing up close. In most cases your brain can adjust to the uneven corrective lenses, and you don't see double. About

70 percent of the people who try this learn to adapt. The success seems to depend on how motivated you are to avoid reading glasses.

Presbyopia usually continues to worsen, requiring periodic changes in your prescription for glasses or contacts. By the time you are about age 65, the lens in your eye has lost its elasticity and doesn't change shape anymore. From this point on you're less likely to need changes in your prescription.

How vision changes with age

As the preceding section on presbyopia indicates, your vision generally changes as you get older. If it doesn't you're a rare exception. Many of the changes are primarily an annoyance. And you learn to adjust to the circumstances. Here are several common changes in the function of your eye:

- Often your retina loses some of its sensitivity to light, so you add brighter lighting to your workstation or near your favorite reading chair.
- Frequently your lenses begin to cloud, causing a decrease in your visual acuity. Colors appear dim, and glare forms when light shines directly at you. This may cause you to avoid night driving.
- Usually your lenses become less elastic and lose their ability to adjust their focus. This may require you to keep changing your reading glasses or to keep a magnifying glass handy for reading small print.
- Sometimes your vitreous shrinks, which may produce bothersome floaters in your visual field. You learn not to let them bother you, although if you notice a sudden increase in the number of floaters, you'll need to contact your eye doctor.
- The conjunctiva and tear glands may lose their ability to properly lubricate your eye. Lubricating artificial tear drops may help correct this problem.

One way to adjust to these changes in your vision is to use corrective lenses. Often by the time you're in your 40s, you'll be wearing some form of corrective lenses, either as eyeglasses or contacts.

Increased risk of diseases and disorders

Although you can adjust to many changes to your vision brought on by aging, some changes can lead to serious eye problems, including partial loss of vision or blindness. Certain vision problems may be an unavoidable, natural part of aging, others can be prevented. Even those that are unavoidable can often be slowed or stopped through early detection and treatment.

Presbyopia, already discussed, is the most common vision problem caused by aging. Other problems include:

Glaucoma. Glaucoma is a condition resulting from abnormally high pressure inside your eyeball. If undetected, abnormally high eye pressure can gradually rob you of your vision — starting with your peripheral vision and eventually leading to blindness. If the disease is diagnosed early, damage from it can be prevented or slowed in most cases with the use of eyedrops. The eyedrops help reduce pressure by reducing fluid production within the eye or increasing the drainage of fluid from the eye.

Cataracts. A cataract is the clouding of your normally clear lens. Almost all of us will have cataracts to some degree as we age. And about half of Americans ages 65 to 75 have cataracts that are cloudy enough to noticeably decrease their vision. Surgery can successfully remove the cataract and replace it with an artificial lens.

Macular degeneration. This condition is caused by a deterioration of the macula, the part of your retina responsible for central vision. Macular degeneration is the leading cause of blindness in Americans older than 65. Some evidence indicates you can take measures to delay development of macular degeneration. There is no treatment for one form of this condition called dry macular degeneration. Surgical treatment is possible for some cases of the other form called wet macular degeneration. The treatment may preserve what's left of your central vision.

Eyelid problems. Eyelid conditions such as entropion, ectropion, dermatochalasis and ptosis may develop due to changes in eyelid tissue or a weakening of eyelid muscles. Any one of these conditions may progress to a point where it irritates the eye or impairs vision. Surgery may become necessary to correct the problem.

Dry eyes. Tears provide an essential lubricant for your eyes. Unfortunately, tear production and tear quality decrease with age, causing symptoms such as stinging, burning and scratchiness in the eyes. Your doctor may suggest a number of steps that you can take to minimize these symptoms.

These conditions, and many more, are discussed in greater detail in later chapters of this book.

Chapter 2

Getting an eye exam

A periodic eye exam is one of the best ways to protect your vision. That's because it's so important to detect eye problems at the earliest stage possible. Several serious eye disorders are capable of doing irreparable damage before they cause any symptoms. If you wait for vision problems to show up before seeing an eye doctor, you may be waiting too long.

A regular exam with an eye specialist helps you:

- Detect eye disease when it's most treatable and before irreparable damage has occurred
- Correct or adapt to vision changes brought on by natural aging
- Reduce eyestrain, fatigue and stress in your daily activities
- Rest assured that you're seeing as well as you can

Who provides eye care?

Three kinds of eye specialists, each with different training and experience, can provide routine eye care: ophthalmologists, optometrists and opticians. Which specialist you choose may be a matter of personal preference. But if you have a serious vision disorder or another health problem that affects your vision such as diabetes, you need to see an ophthalmologist, the eye specialist who has the most medical training.

Ophthalmologists

An ophthalmologist is an eye specialist with an M.D. (doctor of medicine) degree. He or she has a thorough understanding of all serious eye conditions and the treatment options available to you. Like your family physician, ophthalmologists have had at least 4 years of medical school, 1 or more years of general clinical training, and 3 or more years in a hospital-based residency program. They may also have had 1 or more years of training in a subspecialty of ophthalmology.

Many ophthalmologists provide full eye care. They can give you a complete eye exam, prescribe corrective lenses, diagnose complex eye diseases and perform surgery if needed. Other ophthalmologists limit the range of their services. Some offer basic eye care and perform certain surgeries but may refer you to another ophthalmologist for a specialized procedure. Some ophthalmologists perform only selected surgical procedures.

Optometrists

An optometrist can assume many duties of the ophthalmologist. In fact both eye care specialists often compete for the privilege of performing your periodic eye exams. An optometrist, however, stops short of treating complex eye diseases or performing eye surgery.

Optometrists have an O.D. (doctor of optometry) degree. They have usually completed 4 years of training at an optometric school after graduation from college. The schools don't have hospital-based training programs, but some of them collaborate with medical schools to give their students more exposure to clinical practice.

In the past optometrists generally limited themselves to evaluating vision, prescribing corrective lenses and diagnosing eye disorders for referral to an ophthalmologist. More recently optometrists in some states have begun to treat less complicated eye diseases with drugs and perform less complex surgical procedures. In the United States there are almost twice as many practicing optometrists as ophthalmologists.

Opticians

An optician is an eye specialist who fills prescriptions for eyeglasses — assembling, fitting and selling them. Some states also allow opticians to sell and fit contact lenses. The training and licensing of opticians vary from state to state. Most opticians receive on-the-job training with an apprenticeship usually lasting from 2 to 4 years. Some trainees receive classroom instruction as well. Currently only about half the states require opticians to have a license. The American Board of Opticianry and the National Contact Lens Examiners administer tests to certify the skills of opticians.

How often should you have an exam?

How frequently you need an eye exam depends on several factors, including your age, health and risk of developing eye problems. The American Academy of Ophthalmology makes the following recommendations.

Children and adolescents

Children should have their vision tested and be screened for eye disease by a pediatrician, an ophthalmologist or other trained screener. The exams should be done at the following intervals:

- Between birth to 3 months
- Between 6 months and 1 year
- At about 3 years
- At about 5 years

Children and adolescents should be examined whenever they experience any problems with vision or symptoms of eye trouble. The exam should be scheduled as soon as possible. Routine exams are recommended for anyone with a disease that is known to put eyes at risk, such as diabetes.

Adults

If you wear glasses or contacts, have your eyes checked every year. If you don't wear glasses or contacts, experience no symptoms of eye trouble, and are at a low risk of developing eye disease, have a comprehensive eye exam by an ophthalmologist at the following intervals:

- At least once between ages 20 and 39
- Every 2 to 4 years between ages 40 and 64
- Every year or two beginning at age 65

Why do you need exams more often as you get older? It's because of your increased risk of developing an eye disease such as cataracts, glaucoma or macular degeneration.

If you notice any problems with your vision, schedule an appointment with your eye doctor as soon as possible, even if you've recently had an eye exam. Blurred vision, for example, may suggest you need a prescription change. A sudden increase in the number of floaters could suggest vision-threatening changes to the retina.

If you have certain other health problems or a family history of eye disease, you should probably have more frequent eye examinations. Check with your doctor about how often you should be examined if you have any of these risk factors:

- A personal or family history of eye disease.
- A previous eye injury.
- A disease that affects the whole body, such as diabetes, high blood pressure, heart disease or acquired immunodeficiency syndrome (AIDS).
- You were born premature.
- You're black (this increases your risk of developing glaucoma).

The eye exam: What's involved?

When you have a complete eye examination, you undergo a series of tests. The eye doctor will use strange-looking instruments. Bright lights are aimed directly at your eyes. You'll look through a seemingly endless array of lenses. Your eyes may be dilated. Rest assured, each test is necessary and allows your doctor to examine a different aspect of your vision. These aspects include visual acuity, peripheral vision, depth perception, color vision and the ability to focus on close objects. The exam also allows your eye doctor to identify any eye disorders and assess whether damage has occurred.

Questions during the eye exam

If you're seeing a new eye doctor or you have never had an eye exam before, expect someone on the medical staff to ask about your eyes and your medical history. Here is a sampling of the questions:

- Are you having any eye problems now?
- Have you had any eye problems in years past?
- Do you wear glasses or contacts? If so, are you satisfied with them? (Be sure to bring these with you so that the doctor can make sure they're the correct prescription.)
- What health problems have you had in recent years?
- Are you taking any medication? If so, what?
- Do you have any allergies to medications, food or other substances?
- Has anyone in your family had eye problems, such as cataracts or glaucoma?
- Has anyone in your family had diabetes, high blood pressure, heart disease or any other health problems that can affect the whole body?

Visual acuity test

Acuity refers to the sharpness of your vision or how clearly you see an object. Your eye doctor will check how well you read letters from across the room. Your eyes will be tested one at a time, while the other eye is covered. Using the standard Snellen chart, your doctor will determine if you have 20/20 vision.

Your eye doctor may also test how well you read letters close-up by determining the smallest letter you can read on a card held 14 to 16 inches away from your eyes.

Refraction assessment

Refraction refers to how lightwaves are bent as they pass through your cornea and lens. Conditions have to be just right for the light to focus properly on your retina. A refraction assessment helps your doctor determine a corrective lens prescription that will give you the sharpest vision.

Your doctor may use a computerized refractor to measure your eyes and estimate the prescription you need to correct a refractive error. Or he or she may use a technique called retinoscopy. In this procedure the doctor shines a light into your eye and measures the refractive error by evaluating the movement of light that is reflected by your retina.

The eye doctor fine-tunes this refraction assessment by asking you to look through a Phoroptor, a masklike device that contains wheels of different lenses. You'll look at the Snellen chart through various lenses and judge which combination gives you the sharpest vision. By repeating this step several times, your doctor finds the lenses that give you the greatest possible acuity.

Just because the doctor finds lenses that provide you with sharper vision doesn't mean you have to use them. If your uncorrected vision isn't bothering you, there's no need to buy glasses or contacts. Going without glasses or contacts won't make your eyes worse. So don't let any fears about corrective lenses prevent you from getting regular eye exams.

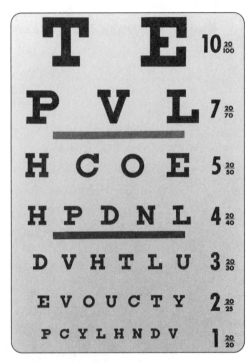

Snellen chart
During a visual acuity test, you are asked to read letters of decreasing size on a chart at a fixed distance from you, usually 20 feet.

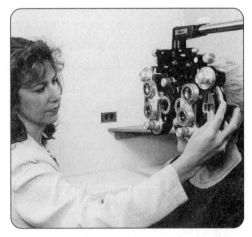

Refraction assessment
A Phoroptor is a device that allows you to view a Snellen chart through different lenses. The lenses are changed until a combination is found that you judge gives you the sharpest vision possible.

Visual field test (perimetry)

Your visual field is the area in front of you that you can see without moving your eyes. In a perimetry test, you look at a testing screen on which a computerized machine flashes spots of light. The flashes will be at different locations on the screen and of varying brightness. Your job is to press a button each time you see a flash. The machine records your responses and maps areas where vision is good. Blank holes or gaps in your field of vision may indicate a serious eye disorder, such as glaucoma or macular degeneration. These disorders, which often develop unnoticed without testing, can be identified by characteristic patterns of visual field loss.

Another test uses the Amsler grid, named after the Swiss ophthalmologist who developed it. The square grid looks like graph paper. In the center of the grid is a black dot (see page 148). Your doctor will cover one of your eyes and ask that you focus the other eye directly on the dot and tell whether you can see the entire grid clearly. You'll need to report if the tiny squares of the grid appear to have different sizes, if any lines look distorted or if part of the graph is missing, as though ripped out by a bullet (see page 143). This will indicate where and to what extent damage to your retina has occurred.

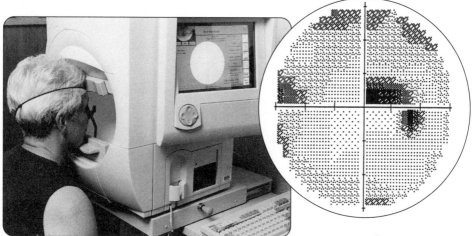

Visual field test

This woman is having a perimetry test done with a computerized machine. The printout (right) shows the visual field of the right eye. The dark area at center right represents a pattern of visual field loss characteristic of glaucoma. The dark area in the lower quadrant is the normal blind spot, representing the optic nerve.

Glaucoma test (tonometry)

By measuring the internal pressure of your eye, your doctor can determine whether you're developing glaucoma, a disease that can eventually produce blindness. If you have glaucoma, the pressure within your eye is usually high.

Two common techniques are used to measure eye pressure. Both measure the amount of force needed to momentarily flatten (applanate) your cornea. With air-puff tonometry the doctor shoots a puff of air at your cornea. With applanation tonometry he or she gently pushes the tip of a tiny, flat-tipped cone against your eye.

A glaucoma test may seem unnerving, but don't worry. It's painless. Thanks to numbing eyedrops applied before the test, you won't feel a thing.

External eye exam

An external eye exam is a quick check of your eyes with no special instruments other than a light. The eye doctor is checking:

- Your pupils to see if they respond normally
- The position and movement of your eyes, eyelids and lashes
- Your cornea and iris for clarity and shininess

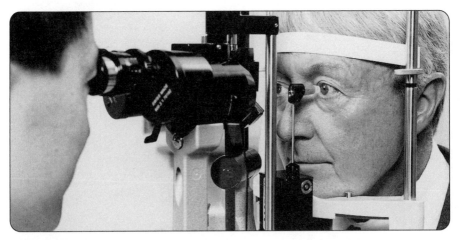

Applanation tonometry
A tiny, flat-tipped cone is mounted on a slit lamp and positioned in front of your eye. By lightly touching the surface of the eye, the doctor measures internal eye pressure. High internal pressure may indicate glaucoma.

Slit-lamp examination

A slit lamp allows the doctor to see the structures at the front of your eye under magnification. The microscope is called a slit lamp because it uses an intense line of light — a slit — to provide oblique illumination of the cornea, iris and lens and of the anterior chamber. The slits allow the doctor to view these structures in cross section and detect any small abnormalities.

When examining corneal problems, your doctor may use fluorescein dye. This dye spreads across your eyes and appears bright yellow when hit with a blue light (screened through a blue filter). This causes tiny cuts, scrapes, tears, foreign material or infections on your cornea to stand out.

Retinal examination

During a retinal examination, the eye doctor puts dilating drops in your eyes to open your pupils wide and provide a bigger window to the back of your eye. Using a slit lamp or ophthalmoscope, he or she can diagnose

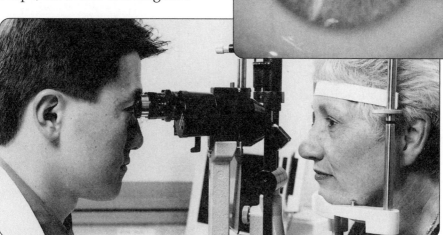

Slit-lamp examination
A slit of light is focused to provide an oblique view of the cornea (arrow A). The crescent of unfocused light on the left indicates the surface of the iris (arrow B). The doctor can also focus this light for a detailed view of the lens.

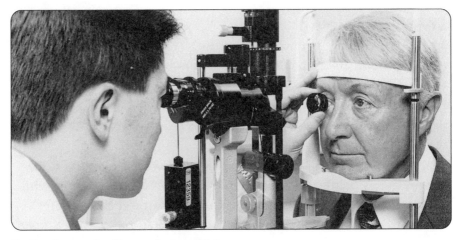

Retinal examination using a slit lamp
The use of a slit lamp, assisted by a magnifying lens held over the dilated eye, gives the eye doctor a clear view of the retina.

abnormalities in the vitreous, the retina, the optic nerve and the choroid. Important clues for the presence of disease elsewhere in the body, such as diabetes and high blood pressure, also can be detected.

Some doctors prefer to look inside your eyes with an instrument called an indirect ophthalmoscope, which uses a bright light mounted on the doctor's head, a bit like a miner's lamp. This lets them see more of the inside of your eye in great detail and in three dimensions.

Dilating drops will usually keep your pupils open for a few hours before gradually wearing off. Until then it will probably be hard for you to

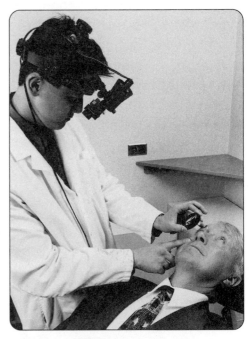

Indirect ophthalmoscopy
With the opthalmoscope mounted on his head and a powerful lens held in front of the eye, this doctor shines a bright light into the eye to examine the entire retina.

focus on close objects. It shouldn't affect your distance vision. With your pupils open this wide, you'll probably need sunglasses for your trip home, especially if it's a bright day. It would be safer to let someone else do the driving.

Fluorescein angiography

Fluorescein angiography is a diagnostic test commonly used for evaluating diseases of the retina and the choroid (see figure 15 in the color section). Fluorescein, a dye also used in checking corneal abnormalities, is injected in an arm vein. As the dye circulates through your eye, the blood vessels in your retina and choroid stand out as bright yellow. A camera takes flash pictures every few seconds for several minutes. These images allow your doctor to assess damage to normal blood vessels and note the formation of abnormal blood vessels. This test is especially helpful for diagnosing and treating macular degeneration and diabetic retinopathy.

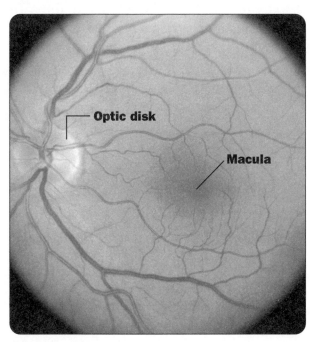

Healthy retina
With a slit lamp or ophthalmoscope, your eye doctor can examine your retina for early indications of eye disorders. A healthy retina should have an even, reddish hue. The optic disk, the macula and the blood vessels that nourish the retina are clearly visible on this image.

Dilated eye examination

A critical part of any eye exam is when your doctor looks at the structures inside your eyeball. Only a thorough examination of the lens and the retina allows the doctor to assess the health of your eye. Many eye disorders are virtually undetectable otherwise, before serious and often irreparable damage has occurred.

Your doctor will put dilating drops in your eye that causes the iris to retract and open your pupil wide. Without these drops the doctor's ability to see the inside of your eyes is seriously hampered. An analogy can be made between the doctor looking through a normal-sized pupil to diagnose eye disease and you peeping through a keyhole to determine all of the contents of a room. Only by opening the door, even a crack, can you truly assess what's inside. In the same way, only by opening the pupil wide can a doctor assess the health of your eye.

Dilation is a safe procedure with few side effects other than blurry vision and sensitivity to light for a few hours until the eyedrops wear off and your pupils return to normal size. While your pupils are dilated, you may not be able to read or do close-up work. You can be prepared by bringing sunglasses with you to wear after the exam. And you can arrange for someone to drive you home.

Chapter 3

Correcting imperfect vision

If you need to sharpen your vision, you have many options to choose from among eyeglasses, contact lenses or the increasingly popular refractive surgery (sometimes referred to as laser vision surgery). A wide variety of lens treatments and eyeglass frames are available — from lightweights for comfort and style to sturdy goggles for playing contact sports. Contact lenses come in rigid and soft styles, which allows you to select a pair that suits your lifestyle and the sensitivity of your eyes. If you prefer not having to deal with corrective lenses at all, you may choose to have your vision corrected surgically. Two surgical options that are especially popular are LASIK and PRK. These acronyms will be explained, along with details of each procedure, later in this chapter.

You and your eye doctor can decide which of these options is best for you. You'll certainly want to take your individual needs into consideration. If your lifestyle or health keeps you from being especially active, glasses may be your best choice. If you're on the go a lot or don't like the look and feel of glasses, you may prefer contacts or the more permanent solution of surgery. Your choices may narrow once you understand a bit about how corrective lenses function and the key differences among the various options.

How corrective lenses correct vision

With normal vision your cornea and lens refract (bend) light that passes through them to focus a sharp image on the retina. If your eyeball is too long or too short from front to back, the image won't be as sharply focused as it should be. The point of focus will lie a little in front of or in back of your retina, blurring the image. A distortion in the curvature of your cornea or lens can also blur vision. For example, the cornea may be more steeply curved from left to right than from top to bottom. The way you can correct these types of vision problems without surgery is by looking through a custom-built lens that compensates for any error in the shape of your eye or the curvature of your cornea or lens. The three basic shapes for corrective lenses are convex, concave and cylindrical.

The refractive power that a corrective lens needs to counteract your specific vision problem is based on the prescription you get from a routine eye exam. The prescription number determines the shape and thickness of your lens. For example, the thickness of a concave lens can vary considerably, depending on whether you are very nearsighted or slightly nearsighted. The higher the prescription number, the stronger the prescription — meaning the more light that must be refracted, the thicker the lens needs to be.

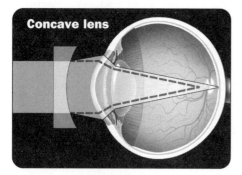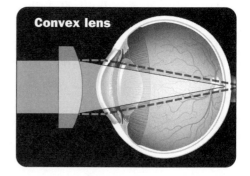

Basic lens shapes
A concave lens (left) corrects for nearsightedness. The dashed lines indicate where the point of focus would be without a corrective lens. A convex lens (right) corrects for far-sightedness and is commonly used in reading glasses. The dashed lines indicate where the point of focus would be without a corrective lens.

Eyeglasses

About 6 out of 10 Americans wear some kind of corrective lenses. And the runaway favorite is eyeglasses. About 8 out of 10 Americans with a prescription for vision correction choose eyeglasses.

The variety of eyeglasses to choose from can seem staggering. Thousands of frame styles and hundreds of lens designs are on the market. And you can buy them from your eye doctor, small optical shops, department stores, discount centers, nationwide optical chains or on the Internet. Eyeglass lenses are made of glass or plastic. Nearly 9 out of 10 eyeglass wearers choose plastic. Once you select the material, you'll be asked to make other eyeglass choices, many of them related to your lifestyle. Your eye doctor can make recommendations if you take a few minutes to discuss the kinds of things you need to be able to do with your glasses. Here are some common lens choices you may need to consider.

Lens materials

Glass. Although glass lenses are usually more scratch resistant than plastic, they can be about twice as heavy. That may be more weight than you're comfortable with, especially if you buy big frames. Another drawback of glass is that it's more prone to break or chip, though it must pass a breakage standard set by the Food and Drug Administration.

High-resin plastic. Costing about the same as glass lenses, these standard plastic lenses are made from a resin called CR-39. They will be a bit thicker than glass but about half the weight. They are also prone to scratching, and for that reason some manufacturers routinely put a scratch-resistant coating on them.

High-index plastic. Lenses made with high-index plastic are lighter and about 20 percent thinner than high-resin plastic lenses. That makes these lenses ideal for moderate or strong prescriptions. Unfortunately, they can cost considerably more than high-resin plastic. They always come with scratch-resistant coating and ultraviolet (UV) light protection.

Polycarbonate plastic. Lenses made from polycarbonate plastic are the strongest available, which makes them the preferred choice for active kids and for use in safety glasses and sports glasses. Though these lenses aren't as lightweight as the high-index lenses, they're lighter than those made of high-resin plastic. They always come with scratch-resistant coating and UV protection.

How to read your eyeglasses prescription

The following example demonstrates how to interpret the numbers and abbreviations of a typical prescription for corrective lenses:

	Sphere	Cylinder	Axis
OD	-2.75	-2.25	90
OS	-1.75	-2.00	90
		+1.50 add	

- **OD** (*oculus dexter*) is your right eye, identified on some prescriptions as RE.
- **OS** (*oculus sinister*) is your left eye, sometimes listed as LE.
- **Sphere** is the correction measurement for your nearsightedness or farsightedness.
- **Cylinder** is the correction measurement for astigmatism.
- **Axis** shows where the astigmatism correction should be on the lens — the position in degrees from horizontal. It can be anywhere from 1 to 180 degrees, with 90 degrees being a vertical (up-and-down) line.
- The term *+1.50 add* at the bottom of the chart refers to an additional lens, in this case, bifocals for close work.

The numbers in the "Sphere" and "Cylinder" columns are units of lens power called diopters, which can increase or decrease in increments of a quarter (.25) diopter. The higher the number, the greater the correction.

A person wearing lenses with the prescription given above is nearsighted, meaning the lenses are concave. That's why the diopters are preceded by a minus sign. On a prescription to correct farsightedness, the numbers would be preceded by a plus sign. The lenses would be convex.

Lens coatings

Scratch protection. A clear, hard coating is applied to lenses to make them more resistant to scratching. In most cases scratch protection is automatically included with high-resin plastic and high-index plastic lenses. Occasionally it's an additional charge. It's a good idea to check that both sides of a lens have been treated because you can accidentally scratch the inside while cleaning it. Be careful where you store your glasses because in extreme temperatures the scratch-protection coating can crack and peel.

UV protection. UV rays may contribute to several age-related eye diseases, such as cataracts and macular degeneration. So when you're outside, it's a good idea to wear glasses that filter out both UVA and UVB light. High-index plastic and polycarbonate plastic lenses will have UV protection. So don't let an unscrupulous or rookie salesperson talk you into paying extra for UV protection that you've already bought.

Antireflection coating. Reflection and glare can make driving difficult, particularly at night. Antireflection (AR) coating helps block the light reflected off surfaces such as pavement, water, snow and glass. This is a big help if you have a stronger prescription, which increases glare. AR coating also reduces the light reflected off your lenses, which makes them nearly invisible. This makes the coating especially useful for public speakers or people who are frequently photographed.

The chemical makeup of this coating makes it harder to keep your lenses clean. And frequent, hard cleaning can rub off the coating. Try to always wipe your lenses carefully with a lint-free cloth moistened with water or a lens cleaning solution. The scratch-resistant coating is generally applied before the antireflection coating, which leaves the AR coating vulnerable to scratches.

Lens treatments

Photochromic. Photochromic lenses are chemically treated so that they automatically adjust to brightness. They get sunglass-dark in direct sunlight and clear in a dimly lit room. They can screen out up to 85 percent of light at their darkest and 10 percent to 15 percent at their lightest.

Some cautions about photochromic lenses: These lenses require UV light to change color, so they won't get dark while you're driving unless the sun is shining on your face through an open window. You may need to keep a pair of sunglasses in the car. Plastic lenses don't change color as quickly or get as dark as treated glass lenses. And neither type of lens changes color as quickly or gets as dark in high temperatures.

Tint. Unlike photochromic lenses that respond to various levels of brightness, tinted lenses remain a constant shade in all situations. Adding color to your glasses can help if you're especially sensitive to light and wish to use your lenses as sunglasses. You may also want to hide wrinkles around your eyes or simply make a fashion statement. Almost any color can be chosen for a tint. Sunglasses are often gray or brown. A yellow tint can make objects appear sharper against a blue or green background.

Plastic lenses are especially adaptable to tints. The lenses are dipped into heated dye to soak up the color. If you want the shade lightened, the tint can be bleached out. Glass lenses, however, are usually tinted by applying a colored covering to the surface. This coating can get scratched off.

Lens edge. If you're very nearsighted, the edges of your concave lens will be thick. This extra bulk can look unattractive and add unnecessary weight to your glasses — especially if you choose frames with large lens holes. A skilled optician can grind the edges so that they blend into the frame.

The frames

When you're looking for new glasses, you may be tempted to start with frames on the display rack. If you want to save time, start with your prescription. Some types of lenses won't work with certain frames. For example, if your prescription calls for thick lenses, a thin wire frame might not be able to support them. A frame with large lens holes may make your glasses too heavy. A skilled optician can tell by your prescription what kinds of frames will work for you, narrowing your search.

Size. The size of your frame can be important for your vision as well as your looks. Some eye doctors think that the frame should cover 20 percent to 30 percent of your face, with the top of the frame following the line of your eyebrows. If your frame is too large, the lenses can pick up too much glare from overhead lights and distort your vision. If the frame is too small, your field of vision may be more limited than you'd like.

If you need strong — and therefore thick — lenses, try smaller frames. They'll reduce the weight of your glasses and may eliminate distortion created when your lenses extend beyond your field of vision.

Materials. Frames come in different grades — or levels of quality — of metal and plastic. Generally you'll get what you pay for. If you buy the least expensive metal or plastic frame, you'll likely get a lower-quality material. Thin metal frames are usually the lightest and most stylish. But plastic frames are usually more durable and better able to support thick lenses.

The cheapest metal frames are made from a mix of metals that include nickel. They may get a coat of color glaze that can peel or flake off in a few months. Some of the cheaper metal frames will corrode from contact with perspiration and salty body oils. This corrosion can damage the frame and irritate or discolor your skin.

The more expensive metal frames made of titanium and carbon-graphite are especially durable. And Flexon, a titanium-based alloy, has "shape memory." You can bend and twist it, and it springs back into shape. The more expensive frames usually get several coats of color glaze. If you live in a warm climate or have a job where you perspire a lot, you might opt for the high-quality metal frames or plastic frames that won't corrode.

Plastic frames, like metal frames, have a range of quality. Propionate plastic is used in the cheaper frames. It doesn't come in a wide range of colors, and these colors are known to fade over time. Zyl plastic is more stylish and colorful but can become brittle. Kevlar, the same strong plastic fiber used for military helmets, is durable. And the newer frames made of a resin called Optyl can be twisted around your finger and snap back into shape.

Fit. If your glasses fit correctly, they'll feel snug and secure, yet they won't rub behind your ears or irritate the bridge of your nose. If the frames do bother you, they can be adjusted at the hinges, bridge or temples — the side arms that rest on your ears. You can also change the tilt of your glasses or adjust them closer to your face.

Your nose supports about 90 percent of the weight of your glasses. So the bridge of your frame is a big factor in determining how comfortable your glasses feel. The saddle bridge is a good choice for heavier glasses. It's a single piece of plastic molded to the frame that sits along the top and sides of your nose like a saddle, evenly spreading the weight of the lenses. The most common bridges are those with adjustable pads, with a pad sitting on each side of your nose. They're flexible and easy to adjust, and the soft silicone material keeps the frames from sliding down your nose.

For active people, such as kids, the temples should hook snugly around the ears and not be so thick that they block vision. Unlike standard hinges that open to a set distance, flexible hinges can hold your glasses tightly to your head but allow the temples to be pulled wider so that the frames slip on or off easily.

After you get new glasses, your eyes and face may need a short adjustment period. This may take a few days or even a week. During this time you may experience some eye ache, but it shouldn't be unbearable or persistent. If it's so painful that you can't wear the glasses, or if the pain lasts more than a week, check with the optician. An adjustment to the frames will probably help. If the pain still persists, ask your eye doctor to check the glasses to make sure the prescription is right. Regardless, it's a good idea to have the fit of your glasses checked every year or so. No matter how well built your glasses are or how careful you are with them, they easily get out of alignment.

Bifocals, trifocals and progressive lenses

Many people use monofocal lenses, which means having only one focal power, to correct for nearsightedness, farsightedness or astigmatism. Other people need multifocal lenses, which combine two or more focal powers in one lens. Chances are that by the time you're in your 40s, you'll need one of the multifocal styles, either bifocal, trifocal or progressive lenses.

It may take practice to adjust to multifocal lenses. But the first step is to make sure the frames are properly adjusted to fit your

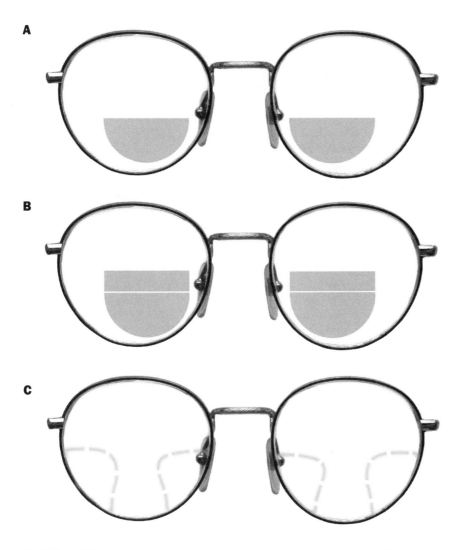

Multifocal lenses

Bifocals (A). As the name implies, the bifocal style combines two focal powers in one lens. The top part of the lens corrects your distance vision, while the lower part (shaded) allows you to read and see objects clearly from a foot or so away.

Trifocals (B). The trifocal lens adds a third power for an intermediate focus between the other two. The added power helps you focus clearly on objects approximately 2 to 4 feet away, such as a computer monitor on a desk, packages on grocery store shelf or books on a library shelf.

Progressive (C). A progressive lens has no division lines in it. Instead the focal powers change smoothly as your eyes move from top to bottom. This means a trifocal, or intermediate, correction is built into the lens. One disadvantage of a progressive lens is that it may distort vision along the bottom edge (dashed line), near the reading section. However, newer lenses have been manufactured with less distortion.

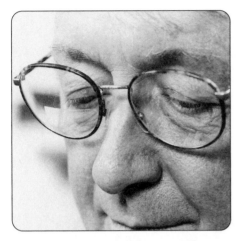 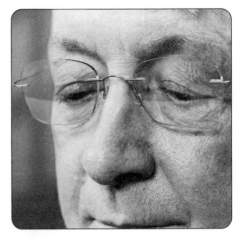

Common designs for multifocal lenses

Flattop semicircle (left). The reading section in bifocals and trifocals appears as a clearly defined semicircle at the bottom of each lens. This design is usually the easiest to adjust to. The line separating the reading correction from the rest of the lens can be polished out so that people don't know you have multifocal glasses. But your vision will be distorted in the small area where one focal power merges into the other.

Executive style (right). Instead of a semicircle, the line dividing the focal powers runs all the way across the lens. This gives you the widest possible field of vision for close work and is often used with trifocals.

head. Tilt your head up and down. Your line of vision should move smoothly from one focal power to the other in both eyes at precisely the same time. Some eye doctors may suggest that you start with progressive lenses, which saves you having to make abrupt adjustments to the different focal powers.

Nonprescription reading glasses

As you enter your 40s, you may find that you need glasses for reading only. You might be able to save money by getting them at a pharmacy or a discount store. Nonprescription reading glasses with lenses of various strengths are often on display alongside the sunglasses. Surprisingly, these reading glasses can also function when worn over contact lenses that correct distance vision.

If your eye doctor has told you the correction for your reading vision, look for lenses of that power. Otherwise use trial and error. The weakest corrective lenses are labeled +1.00, and the strongest are +3.00. Test a few different powers by holding printed material about 14 to 16 inches from your eyes. When you find a pair that allows you to read comfortably, that's probably the power you need. To help you find lenses with the right strength, here's a general guide that shows which power is commonly associated with each of several age ranges:

Ages	Power	Ages	Power
40 to 45	+1.25	55 to 60	+2.00
45 to 50	+1.50	60 to 65	+2.25
50 to 55	+1.75	Over 65	+2.50

You'll need prescription glasses if each of your eyes requires a different lens strength. If you do a lot of reading, you may prefer prescription glasses, which can be more accurate and made of higher-quality material. But the inexpensive glasses made of lower-quality materials won't hurt your eyes. Whether you decide on prescription or nonprescription reading glasses, it's a good idea to see your eye doctor whenever you notice vision changes.

Contact lenses

For some people glasses are a pain. They slide around on your nose. They fly off your face when you're playing hard. They attract dirt like a kid. They need windshield wipers when it rains. They fog up when you come in from the cold. And you're almost certain that someday a mishap is going to fold your $400 pair of glasses into an abstract work of art that's not worth a nickel. Contact lenses are a nice alternative. If you want to wear contacts, the odds are you can. Nine out of 10 people who want to give them a try are able to wear them, including older adults.

Years ago contacts were mainly for nearsighted teens and young adults whose eyes could easily adapt to the hard lenses that were at that time the only type available. But since

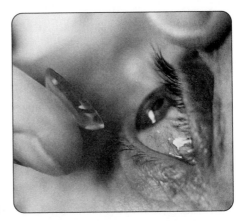

Inserting a soft contact lens

the arrival of soft lenses, which are more comfortable and easier to use, contacts have become more popular with a wider variety of people. About 30 million Americans now wear them. Another reason for the growing popularity of contacts is that now they can correct vision problems that before could be corrected only with eyeglasses. You can even get contact bifocals.

Types of contact lenses

Contact lenses have come a long way since Leonardo da Vinci drew his first sketch of them about 500 years ago, and since a Swiss scientist in 1887 manufactured the first pair out of glass — which, by the way, the human eye couldn't tolerate. It wasn't until the coming of plastics in the 1940s that contacts became practical. The hard contacts developed back then were well tolerated, and the type of plastic used in those lenses is still used today.

Hard contacts. Only about 1 percent of contact wearers still use the original style of hard contacts. These lenses provide sharp vision, but they don't allow oxygen to pass through them to nourish your cornea as well as other types of contacts do. Oxygen gets to the cornea only by going around hard contact lenses. These lenses are also the most difficult to get used to. When you first start using them, you may feel them in your eyes, but your eyes will adapt after several days. Still some people prefer them because hard lenses are the most durable. If you take good care of them, they can last a decade or more.

Rigid gas-permeable lenses. Developed in the late 1970s, rigid gas-permeable lenses are slightly flexible hard contacts that are more porous to oxygen. They offer excellent correction for a wide range of vision problems. They're usually easy to adapt to, comfortable and more durable than soft lenses. For some people "gas-perms" may provide sharper vision than soft contacts. But they have several drawbacks. You have to wear them regularly to keep your eyes used to them. They can slip off the cornea and even pop out of your eye more easily than soft contacts do. And, as with original hard lenses, it's easier for dust to get under them and irritate your eyes.

Soft contacts. Doctors sometimes call soft contacts hydrogels

How to tell if your contact is inside out

Soft lenses sometimes turn inside out. Putting them in and wearing them this way may not affect the sharpness of your vision, but it can irritate your eyes. In fact if your eyes hurt as soon as you insert your contacts, the likelihood is that the contacts are inside out.

There are two ways to check whether a contact is inside out before putting it in your eye. The first way is to hold the lens on the tip of your finger and look closely at the rim. If it's pointing straight up like the edges of a bowl, it's OK. If the edges are flared out, like there's a gnat-sized walking path along the edge, the lens is inside out.

The second way is to put the lens on the crease line in the palm of your hand and gently start to cup your hand. If the edges roll neatly toward each other, like they're forming a tiny taco shell, the lens is right side out. If they start to fold backward, away from the center, the lens is inside out.

because they hold water, which is what makes them so soft and comfortable. The water content varies from about one-third to three-fourths of the lens, depending on the material. Unlike hard lenses, soft contacts allow oxygen to pass through the plastic and nourish your cornea. Softer than rigid gas-permeable lenses, these contacts are even more comfortable and easier to adjust to. But they aren't nearly as durable. Several kinds are available:

Daily wear, or conventional. Daily wear, or conventional, contacts are thin plastic lenses that conform to the shape of your eye. As the name implies, they're designed to be worn when you are awake and taken out before you go to sleep. They're not something you should wear overnight. You'll need to clean them every day you wear them and replace them each year.

Besides being comfortable and easy to get used to, daily wear lenses, like all soft lenses, tend to stay in place. That makes them a good choice if you're involved in sports or are otherwise very active. Like other soft contacts, they can't correct some common vision problems, such as a high degree of astigmatism.

Disposable, or frequent-replacement. Disposable, or frequent-replacement, lenses are thinner and more porous to oxygen than daily wear lenses, which makes them even more comfortable. As the name suggests, disposables are usually worn for a short time and then discarded. Some are designed to be worn only 1 day. Others can be worn during your waking hours for a week or two. Still others can be worn 1 to 3 months. It depends on the design and material and how well you take care of them.

Like other soft lenses, disposables can be harder to handle than hard contacts and can be torn if you handle them too roughly. Also, any lenses that you use for longer than a day need to be cleaned every day. They are prone to surface buildup.

Extended wear. Extended wear lenses are usually disposable and are designed to be worn for more than 24 hours without having to remove them. Because these lenses are designed to provide adequate oxygen to your cornea even while you're sleeping, they're approved for up to 7 days of wear. But most eye doctors don't recommend extended wear contact lenses because regardless of the material they're made of, your eyes receive less oxygen when you sleep while wearing contacts. Furthermore these lenses put you at greater risk of a serious eye infection because the buildup of bacteria on them increases dramatically if you wear them overnight.

Options for contact lens use

To improve or fine-tune your vision, your eye doctor may recommend options other than using a pair of monofocal contact lenses.

Bifocal. Bifocal contact lenses have a reading and distance correction on each lens, like bifocal glasses. The reading section of each lens is weighted, so it stays at the bottom of your cornea and is available when you look down. Sometimes when you blink, the lens can momentarily twist around and blur your vision.

Monovision. With monovision contact lenses, you wear a lens with reading correction in one eye and a lens with distance correction in the other eye (usually your dominant eye). Your brain may adjust to this unequal correction, but your vision will be a bit more blurry than normal. Generally you'll have sharper vision with conventional bifocal contact lenses.

Modified monovision. With this option you wear a bifocal contact lens in your nondominant eye and a contact lens for distance correction in your dominant eye. This allows you to use both eyes for distance, but only one for reading.

Where to get your contact lenses

You can get contact lenses from your eye doctor, a vision care center or even a mail-order business that handles contacts. But first you need a prescription. Contact lens prescriptions are more com-

---

Cleaning your contact lenses

Most eye doctors will give you a starter cleaning kit with your contact lenses. For soft lenses this usually includes a bottle of multipurpose rinsing, cleaning and soaking solution that kills and removes bacterial buildup on your lenses. For rigid gas-permeable lenses, a separate cleaning solution and rinsing-soaking solution is usually needed.

The cleaning kits usually contain instructions on how to use them. Here are some tips that may be useful:

- Before handling your contacts, wash your hands with a mild soap. Avoid creamy soaps that leave a film on your hands, which can transfer to your lenses. Rinse and dry your hands with a lint-free towel.
- Don't use water or saliva to clean your lenses. They contain microorganisms that can cause infection. One particular organism, called Acanthamoeba can cause an incurable infection. Use the sterile cleaning solution your eye doctor recommends.
- For daily wear and rigid gas-permeable lenses, an additional protein-removing enzyme cleaner is recommended.
- With soft contacts some bacteria can penetrate the lenses. So after rubbing each lens in the palm of your hand for a few seconds, soak it in a cleaning solution for at least 4 hours before wearing it again. This kills most of the remaining bacteria.
- Clean your lens case daily with the sterile rinsing solution and let it air dry. Replace the case every 3 months.

plex than those for eyeglasses because contacts require measurements for power, curvature, diameter, and thickness, as well as a selection of design and material. For that reason many states require you to get the prescription from an eye doctor. Others allow opticians to prescribe contacts. A contact lens prescription is determined after an initial evaluation and a follow-up visit or two.

Mail-order businesses can be the least expensive source for contact lenses because of the discount they receive for buying in bulk from the manufacturer. And they pass some of those savings on to you. Most eye doctors offer competitive prices because they aren't trying to make a profit by selling contact lenses. They make their living by taking care of your eyes, providing eye exams and treating eye disorders.

If you get your contact lenses from someone other than your eye doctor, take a couple of precautions.

- Don't continue buying the same lenses based on an old prescription. Get an eye exam every year so that your doctor can check your eyes and see if they've changed. Contact lens complications, if caught early, are usually reversible.
- Don't let the seller talk you into buying a different kind of lens as an approved substitute for the one your doctor recommended. Check with your doctor first.

Refractive surgery

If you're tired of wearing glasses or contact lenses, you may be among the millions of people considering a new and increasingly popular alternative: refractive surgery to correct the curvature of your cornea. The surgery can correct farsightedness, nearsightedness and astigmatism, though it can't help you with presbyopia — the waning of your reading vision that usually starts when you reach your 40s.

In recent years the number of these surgeries has increased annually, from about 400,000 in 1998 to 800,000 in 1999 to about 1,000,000 in 2000. This burst of popularity is due partly to intensive marketing and partly to the surgery's effectiveness — it really does allow many people to get rid of their glasses or contacts. Surgery might be especially attractive if you work in a dusty job and wear contacts, or if you go in and out of doors a lot in cold weather and have to deal with foggy glasses. When swimming or water-skiing, glasses can be impractical or impossible to wear.

Yet this type of surgery has risks. If you're content with your glasses or contacts, you may decide you're better off not taking these risks.

LASIK surgery. About 9 out of 10 people who have refractive surgery will undergo a proven procedure called LASIK, short for laser-assisted in-situ keratomileusis (ker-uh-toe-mi-LOO-sis). This procedure is currently the gold standard for the surgical correction of nearsightedness. The entire surgery takes only 10 to 20 minutes, and the laser beam is generally used less than 1 minute.

Numbing drops are put in your eye. Then the surgeon uses a delicate cutting instrument called a microkeratome to cut a circular flap of tissue from the center of your cornea. This flap, still hinged to your cornea, is about the size and shape of a contact lens. The surgeon folds this flap out of the way and uses a special laser to reshape the layers of your cornea underneath the flap — removing one microscopic layer at a time. A computer, reading a topographical map of your cornea, directs the laser beam to remove tissue where needed.

The laser is known as an excimer laser, or cool laser, because it vaporizes tissue without causing heat damage. Rather it breaks down the molecular bonds. The light beam of energy is absorbed into the tissue being vaporized without harming the nearby lens, iris, retina or other structures of your eye.

If you're nearsighted the laser will trim away layers from the center of your cornea to flatten its dome shape. If you're farsighted the laser will trim away a doughnut-shaped ring to produce a steeper curve. And if you have astigmatism, the laser will smooth out the distortion in your cornea's curvature.

After this brief sculpting, the surgeon returns the corneal flap to its position over the treated area and places a clear shield over your cornea. You wear this shield overnight. The flap quickly reattaches itself to your cornea without stitches.

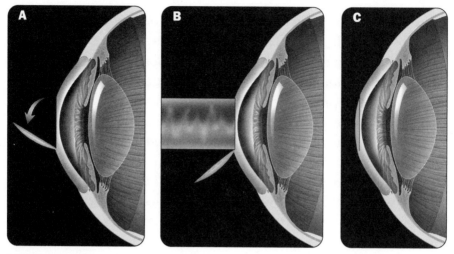

LASIK surgery
A circular flap of tissue is cut from the cornea and folded back (A). An excimer laser reshapes the underlying layer of the cornea (B). When reshaping is complete, the corneal flap is returned to its position over the treated area (C).

Photorefractive keratectomy. Another surgery used with equal success is photorefractive keratectomy (PRK). Instead of sculpting the inner layers of your cornea, the surgeon uses the excimer laser to reshape the outer corneal surface. After removing the thin, protective epithelial layer of the cornea, the surgeon flattens or steepens the corneal curvature. The epithelial layer grows back but conforms to the new shape of the cornea.

With either procedure you can expect to be in the doctor's office about 1 to 2 hours. Follow-up appointments are routinely at 1 day, 1 week, 1 month and 1 year.

Benefits and disadvantages of surgery
Surgery allows about 70 percent of nearsighted people to achieve 20/20 vision without corrective lenses. And more than 90 percent achieve at least 20/40 vision, the vision usually required to pass an eye exam for a driver's license. More recent studies show that these percentages are edging up, a sign of improved technology and surgical skill.

Functional vision — the ability to do most daily activities without corrective lenses — returns in 7 to 10 days after PRK and 1 to 2 days after LASIK. Studies show that by 2 months after surgery, the visual acuity of people who've had PRK is about the same as it is for people who've had LASIK.

When the numbing drops wear off after LASIK, you may feel a sandy sensation in your eyes for a day or so. Yet LASIK is the less painful of the two surgeries because the exposed nerve endings of your cornea are covered by the corneal flap. With PRK the pain can be much more intense, lasting for several days and sometimes requiring powerful painkillers.

After LASIK surgery about 2 percent of recipients don't see as clearly as they did before the procedure. That number drops to 1 percent with PRK surgery. Between 5 percent and 15 percent of recipients eventually need a second surgery to further sharpen or enhance their vision. Other possible problems that may arise after refractive surgery include:
- Increased sensitivity to light
- More problems with glare
- Clouded vision, which typically disappears over time but may continue in some people
- Decreased vision at night, with halos around lights
- Intolerance to contact lenses

The cost is about $1,000 to $2,000 an eye. Usually this cost isn't covered by insurance.

Who's a candidate for refractive surgery?

Typical candidates for LASIK or PRK are healthy adults ages 18 to 55 whose vision hasn't changed in the past year and who have mild to moderate nearsightedness, farsightedness or astigmatism. You may not qualify if you have dry eyes, cataracts, or other eye problems, or if you're pregnant — your vision can change during pregnancy.

Your nearsightedness should be no more than -14.00 diopters (-12.00 for PRK). This can be with or without astigmatism between -.50 and -5.00 diopters (-.75 and -4.00 for PRK). And your farsightedness should be no more than +6.00 diopters.

The surgeon will also want you to have realistic expectations about the procedure, which means knowing the risks and understanding that the surgery may not free you from the need for corrective lenses. Eligibility exams usually require a minimum of 2 hours.

Selecting the right surgeon

You'll want an experienced ophthalmologist doing the surgery —
someone with special training in the procedure, plenty of experience and a high rate of success. Start by asking your primary care
doctor for recommendations.

Once you identify a possible surgeon, ask the following questions. You have only one pair of eyes, so you want to be careful to
whom you entrust them.

- How long have you been doing this kind of surgery? (Look for
  someone with years of experience, not months.)
- About how many of these surgeries have you performed, and
  how many do you do in an average week or month? (You may
  want someone who does some of these surgeries every week
  and who has performed the surgery hundreds of times.)
- What percentage of the people you've treated achieve 20/20
  vision without corrective lenses? What percentage achieve
  20/40 vision? (Look for someone whose numbers are at or
  above the national average of 70 percent for 20/20 vision and
  90 percent for 20/40 vision or better.)
- What percentage of your clients return for an additional
  surgery? (The average is 5 percent to 15 percent.)
- What are the risks and possible complications? (If the doctor
  guarantees the surgery will eliminate your need for glasses or
  contacts, or that the risks are almost nonexistent, look for
  another surgeon. There are no guarantees. And the risks are
  real, with damage that's sometimes irreversible.)

What lies ahead

For those who are weary of corrective lenses that often can't correct
to 20/20 vision, the dwindling risks of surgery and the growing
rate of success makes the procedure all the more attractive. And as
surgical technology continues to improve, along with the skill of
the surgeons, the risks will likely continue to diminish. Some
researchers are anticipating that in the next decade or so, more
detailed computer mapping of the eyes will allow surgeons to
make vision correction even more predictable and accurate.

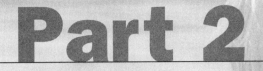

Part 2

Caring for your eyes

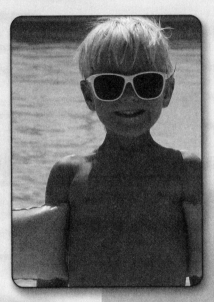

Chapter 4

Protecting your sight

It's easy to take your eyesight for granted. That attitude may change when something happens that hampers your vision. Of course, everyone's vision changes with age and not every eye problem can be avoided. But good eye care goes a long way toward protecting your sight, preventing injuries and reducing your risk of some eye diseases.

What is good eye care? It means wearing protective eyewear in situations that may endanger your eyes. It means developing good habits to avoid eyestrain. It means having your vision checked regularly and keeping chronic medical conditions such as diabetes and high blood pressure under the best possible control. And it's also important to learn to recognize symptoms that may signal a serious eye problem because it may require immediate medical attention. As your mother always said, "Better safe than sorry." It's far better to prevent eye problems than to adapt to life with a vision impairment.

Symptoms that may signal a serious eye problem
- Sudden onset of hazy or blurred vision
- Flashes of light or black spots
- Halos or rainbows around lights

Protective eyewear

One of the most effective ways to protect your vision is to wear safety glasses or goggles in situations that could potentially injure your eyes. According to the National Society to Prevent Blindness, the use of proper eye protection could have prevented nearly 90 percent of all impact injuries to the eye. Many of these injuries happen on the job or during sports and recreational activities. Because sunlight can damage eyes, sunglasses also offer important protection.

At work

Power tools, heavy machinery, potent chemicals — these are among the workplace hazards that can put eyes at risk. Workplace injuries are a leading cause of eye trauma, loss of vision and blindness, according to the American Academy of Ophthalmology. Many workers who have experienced eye injuries had been using inappropriate eyewear or not wearing eye protection at all.

If your job carries a risk of eye injury, your employer is required by law to provide you with safety glasses. Workers in industrial settings, including anyone who works with power tools, are required to wear them. A welder should wear a face shield to filter out the bright ultraviolet (UV) light of a welding arc. Eye protection is also essential on farms, in shops or in laboratories when you work with fertilizers, pesticides, caustic chemicals and solvents.

Around the house

Some of the most common eye injuries occur while people are doing everyday tasks. Spattered cooking grease, splashed detergent or drain cleaner, or sprayed garden chemicals can harm your eyes. So can disinfectants, solvents, oven cleaners, bleach and many other household products. Materials containing ammonia, chlorine, alkali or lye are especially dangerous. When doing hazardous tasks, protect yourself by wearing safety glasses or goggles, and if a child is helping you, make sure he or she wears protective eyewear as well.

If you're working on a car, wear safety goggles to keep rust and other particles from landing in your eyes. It's also a good idea to wear protective eyewear for many other home repair tasks and hobbies.

How to handle an eye emergency

If an eye injury occurs, see an ophthalmologist immediately or go to an urgent care center or hospital emergency room. The full extent of the damage is not always apparent. Even what appears to be a minor injury may cause permanent eye damage if it's not treated.

If you sustain a blunt injury or cut to your eye:

- Cover the eye with some type of shield. For example, tape the bottom of a plastic or foam cup against your eye socket.
- Don't put any ointment or medication in the eye. Don't try to rinse the eye.
- Don't rub the eye. This could tear the tissue, causing more damage.
- Avoid taking aspirin, ibuprofen (Advil, Motrin, others) or other nonsteroidal anti-inflammatory drugs (NSAIDs). They thin the blood and may increase bleeding.

If you get a chemical in your eye:

- Rinse the eye with water to dilute and remove any chemical residue. Try to pull your eyelids open as wide as possible. Flood the eye with a steady stream of water for at least 15 minutes. Tilt your head toward the injured side so that the chemical does not wash into the uninjured eye.
- After rinsing the eye, cover it with a soft pad. Take the chemical container to the emergency room with you, or write the chemical name on a slip of paper and take that.

If you have a foreign object in your eye:

- Don't try to remove anything that's on the cornea or that seems to be stuck or embedded in the white (sclera) of the eye. Don't rub the eye. Cover both eyes with a soft pad.
- If the foreign object is floating on the white of the eye or inside the eyelid, try to remove it with the corner of a clean cloth, a tissue or a cotton swab.

On the playing field

Participating in sports or recreational activities can leave you with more than strained muscles or an occasional bruise. A hard ball or puck hitting your eye at high speed can do serious damage. Finger pokes may scrape or tear your cornea. Physical impact can sometimes break bones near the eye. Water sports may lead to eye irritation or infections. Most of these injuries can be prevented by wearing protective eyewear. Regular eyeglasses and contact lenses aren't enough.

Hard workouts can cause eyewear to fog up. If this happens don't remove your eye protection until there is a break in the action or you have a chance to leave the game. Don't take off your eye protection for any reason during play.

The right gear

Protect yourself by using the right eyewear when playing sports, and if you have children, require them to wear proper eyewear too.

Baseball: a helmet with a polycarbonate face mask when catching; goggles or glasses with polycarbonate lenses on the field

Basketball: goggles with polycarbonate lenses

Football: a helmet with a polycarbonate eye shield and a wire face mask

Ice hockey: a helmet with full face protection approved by the Hockey Equipment Certification Council (HECC) or the Canadian Standards Association (CSA)

Racket sports: goggles with polycarbonate lenses

Soccer: goggles with polycarbonate lenses

Paintball: paintball-specific goggles that meet standard F1776 of the American Society for Testing and Materials

Lacrosse: a helmet with full face protection

Swimming: watertight swimming goggles (Prescription goggles are available.)

In the sun

UV rays from the sun can hurt your eyes as well as your skin. Strong artificial light from sources like welding arcs or tanning lamps can burn the cornea and conjunctiva of your eye much like sunlight can. Long-term exposure to UV radiation can contribute to eye disease, particularly cataracts and age-related macular degeneration.

The best way to protect your eyes from the sun is to wear sunglasses designed to screen UV radiation. Sunglasses don't have to be expensive to be effective. Look for glasses that block 90 percent to 100 percent of both ultraviolet A (UVA) and ultraviolet B (UVB) light. To be even more effective, sunglasses should fit close to your face or have wraparound frames.

Safe fun in the sun

Besides wearing sunglasses, follow these tips to keep your eyes protected in the sun:

- Wear a wide-brimmed hat or cap. Fifty percent of sunlight comes from directly overhead and can slip past most sunglasses.
- Never look at the sun directly, even through sunglasses, because doing so can cause permanent damage to your eyes. You can also hurt your eyes by routinely staring at the sun reflected on water.
- Wear sunscreen on your face and around your eyes, including your eyelids.
- Avoid commercial tanning booths. If you do go, make sure the salon gives you special protective goggles to wear.
- Certain drugs make your eyes more sensitive to light. These photosensitizing drugs include tetracycline (Achromycin V, Sumycin), doxycycline (Doxy 100, Doxy 200, Vibramycin), allopurinol (Aloprim, Zyloprim) and phenothiazine derivatives, such as chlorpromazine (Thorazine) and thioridazine (Mellaril). Wear sunglasses and a hat each time you go outside for as long as you take one of these drugs.
- If you have an eye disease such as macular degeneration, you are at greater risk of UV-related eye damage. Protect your eyes whenever you go outside, no matter how briefly.

Wear sunglasses any time you're outdoors for more than a few minutes. Remember to wear them even on cloudy days because clouds don't block all UV radiation.

You can reduce glare — light that bounces off smooth surfaces such as pavement, water, sand and snow — by choosing darker lenses that block more visible light. Polarized lenses cut reflected glare. But polarization has nothing to do with UV light absorption, so if you're considering buying polarizing glasses, check the label to make sure that they also provide maximum UV protection.

Avoiding eyestrain

Reading in dim light will ruin your eyes, right? Wrong — that's a myth, as is the idea that sitting too close to the TV screen or reading by flashlight will harm your vision. These habits won't do permanent damage to your eyes. But any close-up work, like reading, computer work or crafts, can result in eyestrain. Your eyes may feel dry, irritated, sore or tired. You may have blurred vision, a headache or a sore neck.

Shed some light on the subject
When you're doing close-up work, make sure that you have light well directed at what you're doing. Although a 60-watt to 100-watt light bulb may be sufficient for a person with normal vision, a 150-watt or 200-watt bulb may be needed if you have macular degeneration or reduced vision from other causes. Whenever you change a bulb, make sure the light fixture can handle the wattage of the new bulb.

When reading. When you're reading, position the light source behind you and direct the light onto your page. The light should be bright but not glaring. If you're reading at a desk, use a shaded light positioned in front of you. The shade will keep light from shining in your eyes.

At the computer. When you're working at a computer, place your monitor so that the brightest light source is to the side. Check that the surrounding light is darker than the lightest part of your screen. Position adjustable lighting so that it doesn't shine into your eyes or reflect off the screen.

Glare can be a problem with monitors. The most intense glare will likely come from sources above or behind you, including fluorescent lighting or sunlight. If possible turn off some or all of the overhead lights. Tilting the monitor downward a little, using a glare screen or closing the blinds also may help.

When watching television. Don't totally darken the room when you're watching TV. Instead keep the room softly illuminated. Too great a contrast between the screen and the surrounding area can result in eyestrain.

Combat computer eyestrain

Like many computer users, when you're seated in front of a monitor all day, you may experience eyestrain. Beyond the common symptoms, you may have difficulty shifting your focus between the monitor and the documents on your desk, you may see color fringes or afterimages when you look away from the monitor, and you may have an increased sensitivity to light. Although these symptoms can be unpleasant and disruptive, they won't have long-term consequences. You can relieve or avoid computer eyestrain by changing your work habits and rearranging your workstation and equipment.

Take eye breaks. Look away from the screen and at an object several feet away for 10 seconds every 10 minutes. Or look up from what you're doing and simply let your eyes unfocus. If possible lean back occasionally and close your eyes for a few moments.

Change the pace. Try to move around at least once every 2 hours, giving both your eyes and your body a needed rest. Consider standing while doing noncomputer work.

Blink! Many people blink less than normal when working at the computer. Less blinking means less lubrication from tears, resulting in dry, irritated eyes. Consider using artificial tear drops if you work at a computer for extended periods.

Sit up. Good posture will help prevent muscle soreness in the neck and back.

Adjust your monitor. Position your monitor 20 to 30 inches from your eyes, about an arm's length away. If you find yourself leaning forward to read small type, change to a larger type size or change the page view by zooming in, increasing its actual size.

The top of your screen should be at or below eye level so that you look down slightly at your work. Keep your screen clean. Dust cuts down on contrast and may contribute to glare.

Adjust your keyboard. Put your keyboard directly in front of the monitor. If the keyboard is at an angle or to the side, your eyes may tire from having to constantly move and refocus.

Position reference materials properly. Place books or papers on a copy stand beside your monitor at approximately the same angle and distance away as the monitor.

Wear appropriate glasses, if necessary. If you wear glasses or contacts, make sure the correction is right for computer work. You may need trifocal or progressive lenses to see the screen clearly. Most lenses are fitted for reading print, which you do at a closer distance than the position of your monitor.

Eyedrops

Mild eye discomfort, whether from eyestrain, allergies or other causes, can be soothed with eyedrops. Three types of eyedrops are available without a prescription:

Decongestive eyedrops. Decongestive eyedrops, also called vasoconstrictors, whiten your eyes by shrinking the tiny blood vessels in the conjunctiva. One or two drops in your eye can relieve redness for several hours and often soothe irritation. Improvement should be prompt — if not, see an eye doctor.

Allergy eyedrops. Some decongestive eyedrops include an antihistamine that provides added relief from seasonal allergies such as hay fever. Look for the word *allergy* on the label. Use eyedrops for allergies no more than two or three times a day, unless your doctor gives you other instructions.

Lubricating eyedrops. Lubricating eyedrops, also called artificial tears, contain substances that retain water much like your own

Smoking and eye health

No discussion of good eye care would be complete without mentioning the hazards of smoking. Cigarettes, cigars and pipes were linked to 3,421 eye-related injuries in 1998, according to the Consumer Product Safety Commission. What's more, smoking triples the risk of developing cataracts and macular degeneration, two primary causes of vision loss in older Americans. Finally smoke, like other air pollutants, can irritate the eyes.

tears do. One or two drops of artificial tears can soothe irritated or dry eyes, providing lubrication and comfort. You can use these drops as often as needed.

Words of caution

Eyedrops may contain medicines or chemical preservatives that can cause an allergic reaction. If your eyes or eyelids become even more red, itchy or swollen after you begin using eyedrops, stop using the drops and talk to your eye doctor.

Always use only the recommended dosage of eyedrops. Using some eyedrops more frequently can lead to problems. For example, if you use decongestive eyedrops too often, the redness and irritation may increase after the drops wear off.

If you're at risk of angle-closure glaucoma, don't use eyedrops that contain antihistamines. They can provoke a glaucoma attack.

Putting in eyedrops

To administer eyedrops, tilt your head back and gently pull your lower lid away from the eye to form a pocket. Let the drop fall into the pocket. Don't let the tip of the bottle touch your eye or eyelid. Close your eyes gently and don't blink. Use your index finger to apply pressure at the point where the lids meet the nose. This prevents the drop from draining immediately through the tear duct. Keep your eyes closed for a minute or two. Wipe any excess drops and tears from the closed lids with a tissue. Then open your eyes.

Diet and nutrition

Hardly a week goes by without some new study or book touting the health benefits of various foods. So is there a healthy eye diet? Will certain foods help guard against eye disease? A growing body of evidence suggests that diet can indeed protect your eyesight.

Results published in 2001 from the Age-Related Eye Disease Study (AREDS) showed the impact of dietary supplements on people at high risk of developing the advanced stages of macular degeneration. People in the study group were able to lower this risk by about 25 percent. They also lowered their risk of vision loss due to this disease by about 19 percent. Risk reduction came from a combination of vitamin A (beta carotene), vitamin C, vitamin E, zinc and copper taken in high doses. This dietary supplement did not benefit people in the early stages of macular degeneration, nor did it have an effect on the development of cataracts. Nevertheless here was positive proof of the role dietary supplements can play in preserving your eyesight.

Antioxidants

Vitamin C, vitamin E and carotenoids such as beta carotene, all used in the AREDS, are antioxidants. Antioxidants are vitamins, minerals and enzymes that help maintain healthy cells and tissues. Your body — and your eyes — use antioxidants to combat free radicals when too many are in your bloodstream. Free radicals are unstable oxygen molecules. Normally they perform a number of useful functions. But a surplus of free radicals can damage normal cells in a process called oxidation. Oxidation is thought to play a role in the development of cataracts, macular degeneration and glaucoma, as well as a host of other diseases, including cancer and cardiovascular disease.

Scientists continue to look at the role that antioxidants and antioxidant supplements may play in the prevention of eye disease. Studies suggest that anthocyanin, another antioxidant, may improve night vision and slow macular degeneration. Another study found that people who regularly ate five servings or more of dark green leafy vegetables each week, foods rich in the carotenoids lutein and zeaxanthin, had a markedly lower risk of getting macular degeneration than did study participants who ate smaller amounts or none of these vegetables. At the same time, there's little evidence that taking lutein supplements has a similar benefit.

It will take more research to determine the full effects of antioxidants on eye disease. Reducing risk generally involves including these foods in your diet for many years. Does that mean it's too late for you to benefit from antioxidants? Absolutely not. Including more vegetables and fruits in your diet can't hurt you. And on the chance that they might be protecting your sight, enjoy some spinach or tomatoes today.

Zinc

Zinc is one of the most common trace minerals in your body and is highly concentrated in the retina, although it's not known exactly what role zinc plays in eye function. Some scientists suspect that a lack of zinc may contribute to macular degeneration. A diet with

---

Where to find antioxidants in your food

Vitamin E. Good sources of vitamin E include vegetable oils and products made from them. Wheat germ and nuts also contain relatively high amounts.

Vitamin C. Good sources of vitamin C include green and red peppers, collard greens, broccoli, spinach, tomatoes, potatoes, strawberries, oranges, grapefruits and other citrus fruits.

Carotenoids. Good sources of carotenoids include deep yellow, dark green and red vegetables and fruits, including carrots, winter squash, sweet potatoes, broccoli, bell peppers, tomatoes, papayas, cantaloupe, mangoes, apricots and watermelon. Beta carotene is the best known carotenoid but not the only one. Lutein and zeaxanthin are found in dark green leafy vegetables, including spinach, kale, collard greens, mustard greens, Swiss chard, watercress and parsley. Red peppers and romaine lettuce contain smaller amounts of these two carotenoids.

Anthocyanins. The antioxidant anthocyanin gives the blue color to blueberries and bilberries.

plenty of fruits and vegetables usually provides you with an adequate amount of zinc. If not, you can also take a multivitamin with zinc.

Red wine

Many people who enjoy a glass of wine have been heartened in recent years by studies proclaiming the health benefits of such a practice. For example, a 1998 study suggested that people who drink wine in moderation might be less likely to develop macular degeneration or cardiovascular disease. This benefit may stem from antioxidants found in the wine. Unfortunately the evidence is weak at best, and the conclusions are still premature.

Stick with the basics

The most eye friendly diet is simply a healthy, balanced diet. This should include 5 to 10 servings of fruits and vegetables each day. Look for dark green, deep yellow, or orange fruits and vegetables. You have many to choose from: Swiss chard, bok choy, spinach, cantaloupe, mango, acorn or butternut squash, and sweet potatoes are some examples. Other good choices are vegetables from the cabbage family, including broccoli, Brussels sprouts and cauliflower.

If you eat a well-balanced diet, your body will get all of the nutrients it needs. It's fine to take a daily vitamin and mineral supplement, but remember that supplements are no substitute for eating a variety of healthy foods. Megadoses of vitamins can have dangerous side effects, so stick to the recommended daily requirement listed on the bottle.

Chapter 5

Treating common eye conditions

ost common eye conditions are more bothersome than serious. Your eyes may become red, itchy, irritated, watery, dry or droopy — no fun, to be sure — but with proper care your sight should return to normal. These conditions may involve a doctor visit and, in any case, require following the recommended treatment at home. Several common eye problems are described in this chapter along with guidelines for treating them.

Red or irritated eyes

Exhaustion, eyestrain, lack of sleep or the use of alcohol can turn the conjunctiva of your eye red. The conjunctiva is the clear, delicate membrane that lines the inside of your eyelids and covers the white (sclera) of your eye. If the redness happens only occasionally and clears up quickly, you probably have little to worry about. But persistent redness, especially when accompanied by irritation or pain, can signal a more serious problem.

Conjunctivitis (kun-junk-tih-VI-tis), an inflammation of the conjunctiva, is the most common cause of persistent redness in an eye. Conjunctivitis may be caused by a viral infection, a bacterial infection or an allergic reaction. Viral and bacterial conjunctivitis are common among children and are extremely infectious. Conjunctivitis caused by an allergic reaction stems from exposure to an allergen, a substance that irritates the eye. Allergens and allergen-like substances can be anything from dust or animal fur to spray perfumes, household cleaners or smog.

All forms of conjunctivitis share common symptoms. Most noticeably inflammation causes the small blood vessels of the conjunctiva to become more prominent, giving the normally white sclera of your eye a reddish or pinkish coloration — in fact, one form of this condition is commonly called pinkeye. Your eye often itches. You may notice a gritty feeling in your eye when you blink, as if fine grains of sand were lodged under the eyelids. You may wake up in the morning with your eyelids crusted from mucous discharge. You may have blurred vision and be oversensitive to light.

Conjunctivitis can be an irritating condition, but it's usually harmless to sight and typically doesn't require extensive treatment. Yet because some forms of conjunctivitis are highly contagious, it's important to seek treatment early. If you develop symptoms of conjunctivitis, take steps to prevent the infection from spreading (see "Preventing the spread of conjunctivitis"). Schedule a visit with your doctor. He or she may examine your eyes for swelling and discharge. After learning when and how the symptoms began, your doctor can usually determine what form of conjunctivitis you have.

Viral conjunctivitis, or pinkeye

The viral form of conjunctivitis, known as pinkeye, is familiar to many parents because it's so common among children and can spread quickly through a classroom. Pinkeye may be unpleasant to look at and even more unpleasant to have, but it's usually harmless to sight (see figure 2 in the color section).

Pinkeye typically spreads through contact with contaminated tears or nasal fluids. Symptoms usually appear 7 to 10 days after you've been infected. The disorder often affects one eye first and the other within a few days. Pinkeye produces a watery or mucous discharge. It can develop during or after a cold, and it may be accompanied by a sore throat and swelling of the small lymph glands in front of your ears.

Treatment. Unfortunately, you need to wait for viral conjunctivitis to go away on its own — which usually takes a week or two. Antibiotics won't help this viral infection.

As when you have a cold, get plenty of rest and drink lots of fluids. If the infection doesn't clear up, you may need to consult your doctor. You can soothe the discomfort of conjunctivitis by applying a warm or cold compress to the affected eye. Soak a clean, lint-free cloth in water, squeeze it dry and lay it over your closed eyelids. Artificial tears also may help. You can wipe away any discharge with a moistened, disposable tissue or a clean cotton ball. Wash your hands thoroughly afterward.

Bacterial conjunctivitis
Red, irritated eyes caused by a bacterial infection will produce a

---

Preventing the spread of conjunctivitis

Conjunctivitis caused by viruses or bacteria is highly contagious. Good hygiene is essential for controlling the spread of the disease. Once the infection has been diagnosed, the following steps are useful:

- Keep your hands away from your eyes.
- Wash your hands frequently.
- Dispose of used tissues immediately.
- Change your towel and washcloth daily.
- Wear clothes only once before washing them.
- Change your pillowcase each night. Wash sheets and pillowcases in hot water.
- Discard eye cosmetics, particularly mascara, after a few months. Don't share cosmetics with anyone.
- Discard disposable contact lenses. Don't share contact lenses, lens cleaning solutions or eyedrops with anyone.
- Don't share towels, washcloths, pillowcases, handkerchiefs, glasses or utensils with anyone.
- Stay home from work, school or other community activities until you have no discharge from your eyes. No discharge makes it less likely that you'll infect others.

sticky, yellow-green discharge that may be thicker than the discharge from viral conjunctivitis (see figure 3 in the color section). When you wake up in the morning, your eyes may be matted shut by crusty discharge. Bacterial conjunctivitis comes on quickly, within days of contact. The infection typically starts in one eye and soon spreads to the other.

Many types of bacteria can cause conjunctivitis. And the bacteria can be contracted from many sources, for example, anyone with conjunctivitis or another type of infection. Bacteria can even be spread by someone without conjunctivitis. The germs are passed from person to person through infected body fluids or by hand-to-eye contact. Bacterial conjunctivitis is often associated with a cold. It's common in schools and other places where children congregate.

Treatment. Bacterial conjunctivitis is treated with antibiotics, usually in the form of eyedrops or ointment. For some types of bacteria, antibiotic pills may be given. Antibiotics should clear up the infection within 7 days. It's important to take the medication for as many days as your doctor has prescribed, even if symptoms disappear before the end of the treatment. This will prevent the infection from coming back.

Additional self-care for bacterial conjunctivitis is the same as that for viral conjunctivitis (see page 67).

Allergic conjunctivitis

Allergic conjunctivitis is not an infection. Rather it's a response to an allergen — a substance that can irritate your body. What may be an allergen for you may have no effect on someone else — everyone reacts to allergens differently. Common allergens include pollen, animal hair or dander (skin), dust, chemicals in products such as eyedrops, and some medications. Your body reacts to the allergen by releasing chemicals, such as histamine, that cause the allergy symptoms.

Allergic conjunctivitis, like the viral and bacterial forms, can make your eyes red, swollen and itchy. In addition, your eyes may water, you may have a runny nose, and you may sneeze a lot. It often affects both eyes at once.

Treatment. For conjunctivitis caused by an allergic reaction, treatment may clear up the inflammation quickly, or the symptoms may remain, depending on the allergic trigger. For example, conjunctivitis caused by hay fever can last a whole season and return every year. Treatment may only ease the discomfort.

Medications that may help relieve the symptoms include:

- Decongestive eyedrops can help whiten the eyes, but these drops shouldn't be used for prolonged periods, especially by people with glaucoma. However, a nonsteroidal anti-inflammatory eyedrop such as ketorolac tromethamine (Acular) or diclofenac sodium (Voltaren) is safe if you have glaucoma.
- Allergy eyedrops that contain an antihistamine may help. Mild antihistamine eyedrops are available over-the-counter (OTC), but stronger ones require a prescription.
- OTC antihistamines in tablet form also reduce the discomfort of allergic conjunctivitis.
- Nonsteroidal anti-inflammatory drugs, or NSAIDs (en-SAYDS), such as aspirin and ibuprofen (Advil, Motrin, others) also can help reduce swelling and discomfort.
- Steroid eyedrops may be prescribed for severe allergic conjunctivitis. Steroid drops must be used with caution because prolonged use can cause glaucoma or cataracts.
- Mast cell stabilizers can be used to prevent an allergic reaction. Mast cells, which make histamine, are highly concentrated in the conjunctiva. These medications suppress the release of histamine by preventing allergens from attaching to the mast cells.

Another way to deal with allergic conjunctivitis is to try to stay away from the allergens that trigger your symptoms. If you're allergic to pollen, when pollen levels are high try to stay indoors, keep your doors and windows closed, and use an air conditioner. If you're allergic to animal dander and hair, you may need to avoid pets that shed. If a chemical in a particular eyedrop or contact lens solution causes an allergic reaction, try switching brands.

To ease the discomfort of allergic conjunctivitis, put a warm or cold compress over your eyes several times a day. You can use a washcloth or towel soaked in cold water or wrapped around ice.

Other allergic reactions

Some allergic reactions can be a source of discomfort in the eye without necessarily reddening the conjunctiva. This type of reaction may be a result of common allergens, such as pollen and dust, or of substances that are not true allergens, such as cigarette smoke, perfume and exhaust fumes. Cosmetics also can cause allergic reactions on the sensitive skin near your eye.

In this type of allergic reaction, your eyes become irritated, itchy and watery. The eyelids may be puffy, and dark circles may appear under your eyes. Itchy, scaly, red skin outside the eye and on the eyelid may appear. Though these symptoms can be uncomfortable, they won't permanently hinder your sight. You might be tempted to rub your eyes, but doing so will just cause more irritation and itching.

Treatment. The treatment for allergic reactions in the eye is the same as that for allergic conjunctivitis. For many people an antihistamine eyedrop or tablet will provide sufficient relief and comfort.

To treat an allergic reaction on the skin around your eyes, apply a cold compress to the affected area four or more times a day to decrease swelling. You can also take antihistamine tablets. In severe cases your doctor might prescribe a steroid cream or ointment for use near the eye.

What's that red spot in my eye?

Have you ever been alarmed to discover a bright red patch on your eye? This scary-looking spot is usually a subconjunctival hemorrhage (see figure 4 in the color section). It happens when a blood vessel in the conjunctiva breaks, leaking blood into the thin space between the conjunctiva and the white of the eye (sclera). The blood vessel may break for no reason at all or when you cough, sneeze or vomit forcefully. An injury to the eye also can cause such a hemorrhage.

If you have pain with a broken blood vessel or if you get them recurrently, contact your doctor. Otherwise a subconjunctival hemorrhage doesn't require treatment. The red spot will go away after several days.

Eyelid-related problems

The eyelids are extremely important protectors of your eyes. Quick, powerful reflexes make the eyelids close when an object nears or when irritating particles are in the air. The eyelids lubricate your eyes and wipe foreign particles from them. Occasionally the eyelids can be the site of problems.

Sties and other eyelid swellings

A sty (hordeolum) is a red lump on the edge of your eyelid that may resemble a boil or a pimple (see figure 5 in the color section). It stems from a bacterial infection near the root of an eyelash. A sty develops over several days. It fills with pus and becomes painful to touch but is usually harmless to the eye.

Another form of swelling on the eyelid is a chalazion (kuh-LAY-ze-on). Unlike a sty it develops a little farther up and within the eyelid (see figure 6 in the color section). It's not an infection but a swelling caused by blockage of one of the small oil glands that help lubricate the eye. A chalazion is relatively painless but may be unsightly.

Treatment. About a week after it first appears, a sty usually ruptures, which relieves the pain. The swelling will go down in another week or so. Begin using a clean, warm compress as soon as you feel a sty coming on. Apply the compress four times a day for 10 minutes until the sty opens. Don't squeeze it in an effort to remove the pus — let the sty burst on its own. Once the sty has opened, wash your eyelid thoroughly to prevent the bacteria from spreading.

Consult your doctor if the sty interferes with your vision, does not disappear on its own or is recurring. A particularly stubborn sty may need to be lanced and drained. If you're prone to recurring sties, your doctor may prescribe an oral antibiotic.

A chalazion will often go away without treatment, although how long that takes may vary from 1 to 2 weeks. Applying a warm compress to it four times a day for 10 minutes will help. You can also massage the area four times a day to break up the lump. If a chalazion gets big enough to affect your vision, your doctor may inject it with a steroid solution or lance it and drain the swelling.

If you have recurring chalazions, your doctor may want to do a biopsy, removing a small sample of tissue to see if the lump is a cancerous tumor.

Blepharitis

Blepharitis (blef-uh-RI-tis) is an inflammation of the eyelids along their edges (see figure 7 in the color section). Some people produce excess oil in glands near their eyelashes. The oil encourages the growth of bacteria, which can make the eyelids irritated and itchy. Blepharitis is often a chronic condition that involves seborrheic dermatitis, which is the abnormal secretion of oil in the skin, particularly around the scalp and face. People with rosacea, dandruff or dry eyes are also likely to get blepharitis. Although it's uncomfortable and not very attractive, blepharitis doesn't cause permanent damage to sight.

Signs and symptoms of blepharitis can also include a gritty, burning sensation in your eyes, watery or red eyes, swollen eyelids, and flaking of the skin around the eyes. The eyelids may appear greasy and crusted with scales that cling to the lashes. This debris can cause the eyelids to stick together at night. Don't be concerned if you have to pry your eyes open in the morning because of these sticky secretions.

Treatment. The key to treating chronic eyelid inflammation is good hygiene. This alone may allow you to control symptoms and prevent complications.

Follow this self-care remedy one to two times a day:

1. Apply a warm compress over your closed eyes for 10 minutes.
2. Immediately afterward use a washcloth moistened with warm water and a few drops of baby shampoo to wash away any oily debris and scales at the base of the eyelashes.
3. Rinse the lids with warm water and gently pat them dry with a clean, dry towel.

Continue this treatment until your symptoms disappear. If your condition doesn't improve, contact your doctor. He or she may prescribe an antibiotic cream, an antibiotic ointment or, in severe cases, eyedrops containing antibiotics and steroids.

Figure 1a. Front of the eye

The light that enters the front of your eye is a continuous information stream, providing vast amounts of data about the world for you to process and analyze. Your perception of color and movement and your ability to judge speed, distance and depth depend on eyesight. Vision supports your interactions and emotional connections with others. Vision works with your other senses to sharpen the experience of living. For example, your senses — vision, taste and smell in particular — interact to enhance your enjoyment of a good meal.

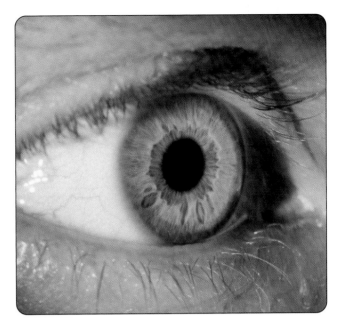

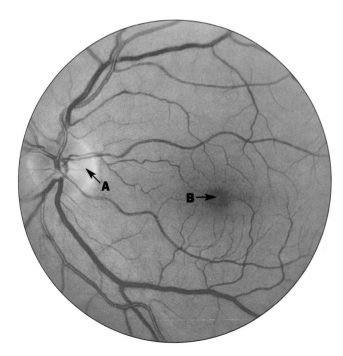

Figure 1b. Back of the eye

The retina (as viewed through an ophthalmoscope) is a layer of tissue at the back of the eye, consisting of millions of light-sensitive cells and other nerve cells. The retina captures the data carried by light and relays it to the visual cortex, the seeing portion of your brain. A healthy retina has an even, reddish hue. The optic disk is the yellowish-orange structure with blood vessels radiating from it (arrow A). The macula is the deep red spot at the center of the retina (arrow B).

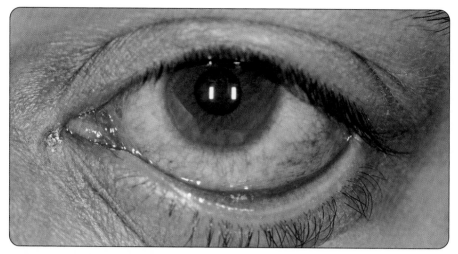

Figure 2. Viral conjunctivitis
Viral infection of the conjunctiva engorges blood vessels of the eye, giving it a swollen, red and teary appearance.

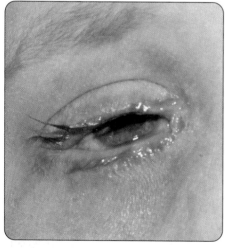

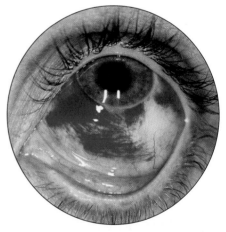

Figure 4. Subconjunctival hemorrhage
When a small blood vessel breaks in the conjunctiva, blood accumulates in this blotchy fashion. It may look scary, but this condition is harmless and usually disappears in a few days.

Figure 3. Bacterial conjunctivitis
Bacterial conjunctivitis not only causes redness and swelling but also often produces a thicker mucous discharge than does viral conjunctivitis.

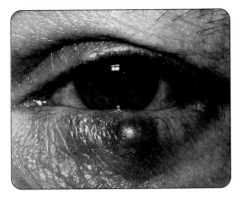

Figure 5. Sty
A sty is a painful, reddish swelling caused by a bacterial infection along the edge of your eyelid.

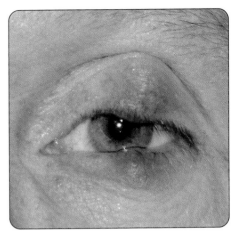

Figure 6. Chalazion
A chalazion (on the upper eyelid) is a relatively painless swelling caused by inflammation, usually located away from the edge of your eyelid. (A sty is located on the lower eyelid.)

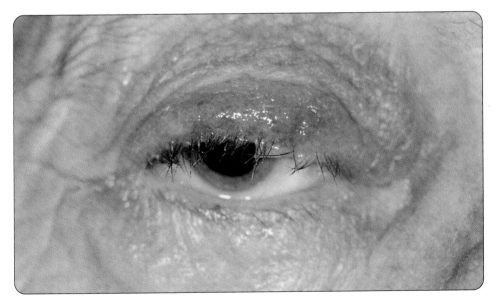

Figure 7. Blepharitis
An eyelid with blepharitis may appear red and swollen with scaly, greasy debris along the lid margin. Blepharitis is often associated with dandruff of the scalp and the eyebrows.

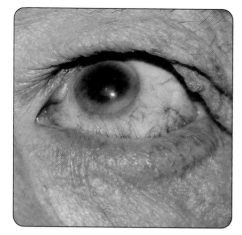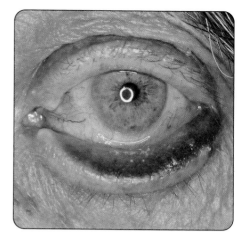

Figure 8. Entropion and ectropion
With entropion (left) the eyelid turns inward, allowing the lashes to rub against and irritate the eyeball. With ectropion (right) the eyelid sags away from the eyeball. Lacking protection and sufficient lubrication, the eye becomes red and irritated.

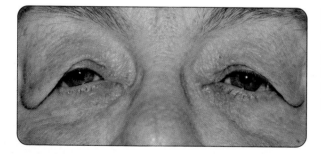

Figure 9. Dermatochalasis
A relaxation of the skin of the upper eyelid may cause it to droop over the eyelashes and interfere with your vision.

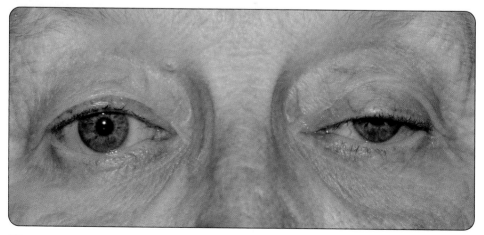

Figure 10. Ptosis
A weakening of the muscle that raises the upper eyelid can cause the entire lid to droop over the eye (right).

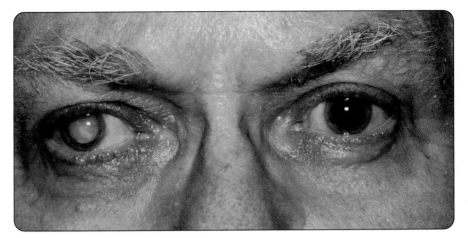

Figure 11. Cataract

The lens of the eye (left) has become cloudy, giving the pupil a white appearance.

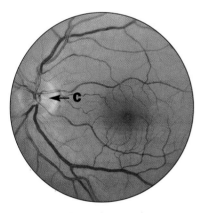

Figure 12. Glaucoma

In the image on the right, the optic nerve has been affected by advanced glaucoma. This is evident from the excavation, or cupping, at the center of the optic disk (arrow A). Only a narrow rim of optic nerve tissue around the edge remains (arrow B).

In comparison, the optic disk of a healthy eye (above) has more even and reddish coloration (arrow C).

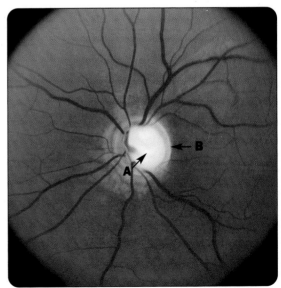

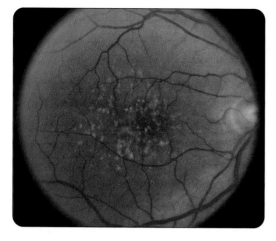

Figure 13. Early-stage dry macular degeneration

The hallmark of early-stage dry macular degeneration is the appearance of drusen in and around the macula. Drusen, which are waste deposits, look like yellow spots under the retina.

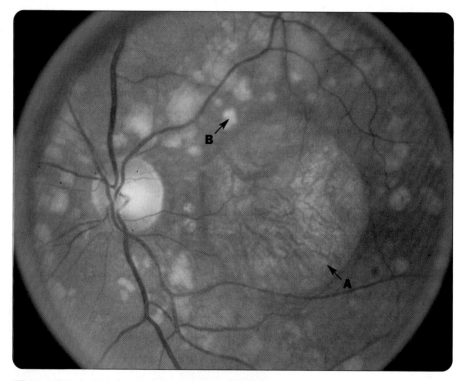

Figure 14. Late-stage dry macular degeneration

The retinal pigment epithelium at the center of the retina has disappeared, exposing the blood vessels of the choroid that lie underneath the macula (arrow A). Large drusen (such as the one indicated by arrow B) surround the macula.

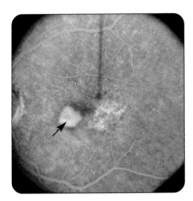

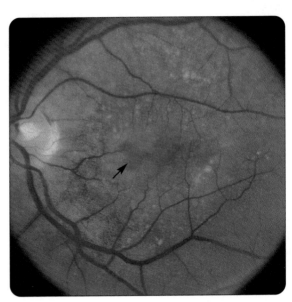

Figure 15. Wet macular degeneration

In wet macular degeneration, abnormal blood vessels develop under the retina (see arrow at right). A fluorescein angiogram of the same eye allows the doctor to accurately detect these abnormal blood vessels (see arrow above).

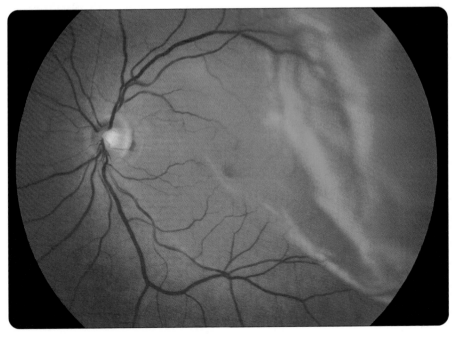

Figure 16. Retinal detachment

A section of the retina is gray and folded on the upper right where it has separated (detached) from the inside wall of the eye.

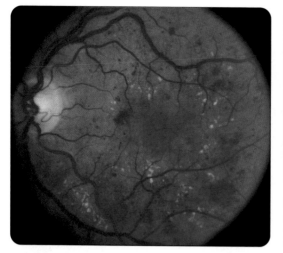

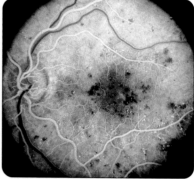

Figure 18. Fluorescein angiogram of diabetic retinopathy

This image (the same eye as in figure 17) shows numerous microaneurysms as intense white dots. The dark spots are hemorrhages and fatty deposits (exudates).

Figure 17. Nonproliferative diabetic retinopathy

Engorged blood vessels, microaneurysms (tiny red dots), hemorrhages (large red blots) and fatty deposits, or exudates (yellow spots), are the most commonly observed signs of nonproliferative diabetic retinopathy.

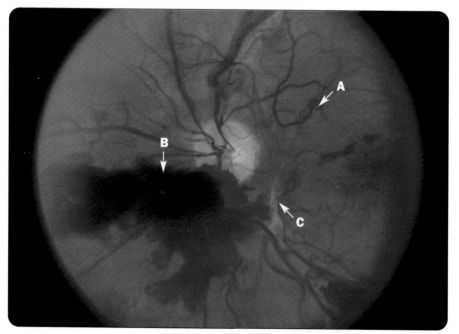

Figure 19. Late-stage proliferative diabetic retinopathy

In proliferative diabetic retinopathy, abnormal blood vessels grow on the optic nerve and the retina and into the vitreous cavity (arrow A). These blood vessels break, causing vitreous hemorrhages (arrow B) and the formation of scar tissue (arrow C).

A twitchy eyelid

From time to time your eyelid may take on a life of its own, twitching at random. This involuntary quivering of the eyelid muscle usually lasts less than a minute, but it can drive you crazy and make you wonder if something's wrong with your eyes.

A twitch is usually harmless. You may be able to relieve the twitching by gently massaging the affected eyelid. The cause of the twitching is unknown, but the condition is often associated with fatigue and stress. Rarely a twitching eyelid is a symptom of a muscle or nerve disease, but the twitching is usually accompanied by other symptoms.

Entropion

With entropion the eyelid — usually the lower lid — turns in toward the eye, allowing the skin of the eyelid and the eyelashes to rub against the conjunctiva (see figure 8 in the color section). In addition to eye irritation, entropion can cause excessive tearing, discharge, crusting of the eyelid and a feeling that something is lodged in the eye. In severe cases the turned-in lashes may scratch the cornea, resulting in an infection or scarring of the cornea and impaired vision.

Most often entropion develops when the tissues of the eyelid relax as a result of aging. One of the first signs of the condition is irritation of the eyes in the morning, which usually clears later in the day. As the disorder advances, the irritation may become more frequent, even constant. You may notice the lashes turning in toward the eye, especially when you blink forcibly.

Treatment. Artificial tears or lubricating ointment can offer temporary relief for entropion by providing additional moisture. Some people wear a plastic eye shield at night to retain moisture.

The primary means of treating this condition is surgery to reposition the eyelid. The doctor does this by adjusting muscles or tendons of the eyelid. This is a fairly simple procedure that's usually performed on an outpatient basis using a local anesthetic. After surgery you may wear an eye patch overnight and use an antibiotic ointment for about a week.

Ectropion

Ectropion, like entropion, involves the eyelid, usually the lower lid. But with ectropion the eyelid turns out, rather than in, and sags (see figure 8 in the color section). The eyelid can no longer close properly, and without the protection of the lid, the inside of the eyelid and the surface of the eye become dry, irritated and inflamed. Normal tears flow out instead of lubricating the eye. Rubbing the eye can lead to encrusted eyelids and mucous discharge.

Ectropion is most often due to relaxation of the muscles and tendons in the eyelid as a result of aging. The condition can also be caused by scarred lid tissue from burns, trauma, tumors, a facial nerve disorder or previous eyelid surgery. Untreated ectropion can lead to infection, damage to the cornea from exposure and inadequate lubrication, and ultimately impaired vision.

Treatment. The treatment for ectropion is much the same as that for entropion (see page 73). In addition some people tape the sagging lid in place at night to keep it from turning outward.

Dermatochalasis

As you age your eyelid skin gradually begins to stretch and sag. Fat gathers over and under the eyes. This age-related drooping of the skin in the upper or lower eyelid is called dermatochalasis (dur-muh-toe-KAL-uh-sis) — see figure 9 in the color section. In the upper eyelid, this condition may cause the eyelid skin to sag over your eyelashes and interfere with vision. The lower eyelid may form what is commonly known as bags under your eyes. Dermatochalasis usually affects both eyes.

Treatment. A surgical procedure called blepharoplasty (BLEF-uh-ro-plas-te) is commonly performed to remove excess skin, muscle and fat from the eyelid. It's generally a safe procedure and can be done on an outpatient basis. Blepharoplasty shouldn't interfere with your vision, and any swelling, tenderness or pain you experience afterward should subside in 2 to 4 weeks. Mild cases of dermatochalasis are sometimes treated with laser surgery. In this procedure skin and muscle are shrunk and tightened rather than removed.

Whether your insurer will pay for blepharoplasty depends on

whether the drooping eyelid impairs your vision. Most insurers, including Medicare, don't cover surgery done strictly for cosmetic reasons but may pay if the sagging skin interferes with eyesight. To assist you, your doctor may conduct tests to document your vision impairment due to the drooping eyelid before surgery.

Ptosis

Less common and more complicated than dermatochalasis is a condition called ptosis (TOE-sis) — see figure 10 in the color section. It's caused by a weakness of the muscle that raises the upper eyelid and keeps it in an open position. Whereas dermatochalasis results in sagging eyelid skin, ptosis causes the entire lid to droop. Ptosis can affect one or both eyes and may partially block vision.

Ptosis often runs in families. Some children are born with ptosis, usually in one eye only. In adults ptosis can be a result of aging or an injury. A condition affecting nerve and muscle response, such as myasthenia gravis, stroke, diabetes or a brain tumor, can also cause ptosis. A drooping eyelid that develops suddenly requires immediate attention. It may be a sign of stroke or another acute problem within your nervous system.

Treatment. If eyelid droop affects your vision, a thorough eye examination may be necessary to determine the cause. If the drooping is due to a nerve or muscle condition, treating this underlying cause may improve the ptosis. If the drooping is the result of aging or injury, your eye doctor may perform an operation to strengthen the muscle. This surgery may involve shortening the eyelid muscle and removing some of the overlying skin. It's a complicated operation that should be performed by a specialist in this type of surgery.

Tear-related problems

A sad movie or a wedding can make your tears flow. But expressing emotion is just one of the many functions of tears. Tears protect the eyes and lubricate them, an essential part of clear, comfortable vision. Tears reduce the risk of eye infection and, with each blink of the eyelid, help clear the eye of any debris. When your eyes become irritated from dust or are bothered by wind, smoke or fumes, extra tears form to help wash away the foreign material.

There are many other causes of watery eyes, including allergic reaction, sinus infection, eye infections and nasal problems. Ironically, dry eyes often produce excess tearing (see "If my eyes are dry, why are they watering?" on page 80). Occasionally tear duct problems result in continuously watering eyes.

Blocked tear duct

The tear-producing glands, called the lacrimal glands, are located under the brow bone, just above your eyes. When you blink, your upper eyelids spread tears over the surface of your eyes and pump excess fluid into ducts that drain to your nose. That's why your nose often runs when you cry. If a tear duct (lacrimal duct) becomes blocked, fluid backs up and spills over the eyelid, causing tears to run down your cheek.

Tear duct blockage is rare, but it can be associated with aging, inflammation of a nasal passage or injury to the nose. Usually only one eye is affected. About 5 percent of babies are born with a blocked tear duct. This congenital blockage often disappears on its own within 6 months.

A blocked tear duct can become infected from bacteria in the stagnant tears. This condition is called dacryocystitis (dak-re-o-sis-TI-tis). Tissue between the inner angle of the eye and the bridge of the nose becomes swollen and tender.

Treatment. If your eye waters constantly over a period of several days, see an eye doctor. If the problem is a blocked duct, the doctor may probe and

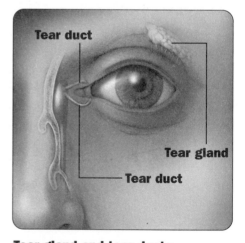

Tear duct

Tear gland

Tear duct

Tear gland and tear ducts
The tear gland, located above each eyeball, continuously supplies tear fluid that is distributed by the action of your blinking eyelids. Excess fluid drains through the tear ducts into the nose.

flush (irrigate) the tear duct to help diagnose your condition. This is a simple outpatient procedure. Applying a warm compress to the eye several times a day can help relieve the discomfort. Your doctor may also prescribe antibiotics.

If your symptoms are severe and don't improve, your doctor may recommend surgery to create a new tear duct. In this operation, the doctor may use thin silicone tubing to keep the new tear duct open while healing occurs.

In rare cases the blockage is beyond repair, and it's necessary to surgically implant an artificial tear duct. The artificial duct, called a Jones tube, is made of unbreakable glass and placed in the inner corner of the eyelid.

Dry eyes

Dry eyes occur when the system that produces your tears breaks down. This causes the cornea, or parts of it, to dry out. Symptoms include a stinging, burning, or scratchy sensation, stringy mucus in or around the eyes, increased eye irritation from smoke or wind, eye fatigue after short periods of reading, and difficulty wearing contact lenses. Both eyes are usually affected.

Some people don't produce enough tears to keep their eyes comfortably lubricated. This may be due to aging, medications, menopause, autoimmune disorders, chemical burns or eyelid deformities. Other people produce a normal amount of tears, but the composition of the tears is of poor quality. That means the tears lack certain components, such as oil, that are essential for lubrication. Problems unrelated to tear production may also cause eyes to feel dry and scratchy. These include:

- Blepharitis
- Entropion or ectropion
- Environmental irritants such as smoke, sun, wind and indoor heating
- Disruption of your blink reflex
- An allergic reaction to eyedrops or ointment
- Eyestrain

Although dry eyes don't usually cause permanent damage, diminished vision may prompt people to seek medical treatment.

Medications and dry eyes

A wide variety of common medications, both prescription and over-the-counter (OTC), can cause dry eyes. These include:

- Diuretics
- Antihistamines and decongestants
- Sleeping pills
- Tricyclic antidepressants
- Accutane-type drugs for treatment of acne
- Opiate-based pain relievers such as morphine

Decreased tear production. Like skin and hair, your tear production tends to dry up as you get older. When you're unable to produce enough tears, your eyes become easily irritated. The medical term for this condition is *keratoconjunctivitis sicca* (ker-uh-to-kun-junk-ti-VIE-tis sik-uh).

Although dry eyes can affect both men and women at any age, it is more common among women, especially after menopause. This may be due to hormonal changes brought on by this phase. Damage to the lacrimal glands from inflammation or radiation can hamper tear production. Dry eye is also associated with medical conditions such as rheumatoid arthritis, systemic lupus erythematosus (SLE), scleroderma and Sjogren's syndrome.

Poor tear quality. Tears are much more than just water. They are a complex mixture of water, fatty oils, proteins, electrolytes, bacteria-fighting substances and growth factors that regulate various cell processes. This mixture helps make the eye surface smooth and clear. Without it good vision is impossible.

The eyelids spread tears across the surface of the eye in a thin film. The tear film has three basic layers:

Mucus. The inner layer consists of mucus produced by the conjunctiva. This layer allows tears to spread evenly over the surface of the eye.

Water. The middle layer, which makes up about 90 percent of the tear, is mostly water with a little bit of salt. This layer, produced by the lacrimal glands, cleanses the eye and washes away foreign particles or irritants.

Oil. The outer layer, produced by glands on the edge of the eyelid, contains fatty oils called lipids. These smooth the tear surface and slow evaporation of the watery layer.

Considering this complicated mix of ingredients, it's not surprising that the balance is sometimes off. An imbalance causes the tears to evaporate faster and your eyes to become dry. Certain diseases or chemical burns can cause changes in the oily and mucous layers of your tears. Blepharitis, rosacea and other skin disorders also can disrupt production of the oily layer.

Treatment. If your eyes feel dry and irritated, your eye doctor can test both the quantity and quality of your tears. The doctor may measure your tear production using the Schirmer tear test. In this test blotting strips of paper are placed under the lower eyelids. After 5 minutes the amount of strip soaked by the tears is measured.

Other tests use special dyes in eyedrops to determine the surface condition of your eye. The doctor looks for staining patterns on the cornea and measures how long it takes before your tears evaporate.

Regardless of the cause of dry eyes, the goal of treatment is to keep your eyes moist. This can be done either by replacing the tears or conserving them.

Adding tears. A mild case of dry eyes usually can be treated with artificial tears. You can use the lubricating drops as often as needed, even several times an hour, to provide relief. If you use drops frequently, preservative-free eyedrops might be the best choice to avoid an allergic or toxic reaction to preservatives. People with dry eye disorders are often more prone to irritation from preservatives in eyedrops.

Ointments can be used to ensure lubrication. These ointments can blur vision, so it's best to use them only at night.

Conserving tears. Your eye doctor may also suggest methods to keep your tears from draining. The tear drainage ducts can be plugged either temporarily or permanently with tiny collagen or silicone plugs. The closure conserves both your own tears and artificial tears you may have added. Collagen plugs will slowly dissolve over a few days. Silicone plugs can be removed or left in. A more permanent option is thermal cautery. In this procedure the doctor numbs the area with an anesthetic and then applies a hot

If my eyes are dry, why are they watering?

It sounds like a contradiction, but you may have dry eyes and still at times find yourself with tears streaming down your cheeks. Why?

Tears are produced in two ways. Basic tearing produces tears at a slow, steady rate and keeps the eyes lubricated. What's called reflex tearing produces large quantities of tears in response to eye irritation or emotions. Reflex tears contain much more water than do basic tears, and they're low in mucus and oils.

When your eyes become irritated from dryness, the lacrimal gland floods the eye with reflex tears. Fluid overwhelms the tear duct and overflows your eyelids. What's more, because these tears are of poor quality, they don't help the dryness. That may make you produce even more tears.

wire that shrinks the tissues of the drainage area and causes scarring, which closes the tear duct.

Anti-inflammatory drugs. Some evidence suggests that the underlying cause of dry eyes is an inflammation in the lacrimal glands and on the surface of the eye. For this reason researchers are investigating anti-inflammatory drugs for treating dry eyes. The results of one clinical trial suggested that people who received such a drug, cyclosporine A, experienced significant improvement in their dry eye symptoms with few side effects. When people experience intolerable irritation from dry eyes despite the frequent use of lubricating eyedrops, doctors may prescribe steroid drops.

Self-care. Like any liquid, tears will evaporate when exposed to air. These are simple steps you can take to help slow evaporation:

- Don't direct hair dryers, car heaters, air conditioners or fans toward your eyes.
- Wear glasses on windy days and goggles while swimming.
- Keep your home humidity between 30 percent and 50 percent. In winter a humidifier can add moisture to dry indoor air.
- Remember to blink. Consciously blinking repeatedly helps spread your own tears more evenly.

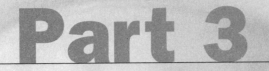

Part 3

Eye diseases and disorders

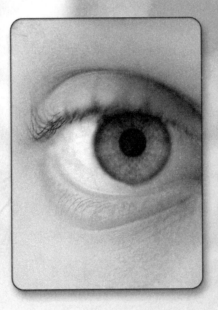

Chapter 6

Glaucoma

Glaucoma is sometimes called the silent thief, slowly stealing your sight before you realize anything's wrong. The most common form of glaucoma develops gradually, giving no warning signs. Many people aren't even aware they have an eye problem until their vision is extensively damaged. Glaucoma is the second most common cause of vision loss in the United States. It affects approximately 3 million Americans.

Actually, glaucoma is not just one disease but a group of them. The common feature of these diseases is that abnormally high pressure inside the eyeball damages the optic nerve. The optic nerve is a bundle of more than a million nerve fibers at the back of the eye. It's like a big electric cable made up of thousands of individual wires carrying the images you see from the retina to the brain. Blind spots develop in your visual field when the optic nerve deteriorates, starting with your peripheral (side) vision. If left untreated glaucoma may lead to blindness in both eyes.

Fortunately, only a small percentage of people with the disease ever lose their sight. Recent medical advances have made it easier to diagnose and treat glaucoma. And if detected and treated early, glaucoma need not cause even moderate vision loss. But it does require regular monitoring and treatment for the rest of your life.

Understanding eye pressure

Internal pressure in your eye, called intraocular pressure (IOP), allows the eye to hold its shape and function properly. IOP is like air in a balloon — too much pressure inside the balloon affects its shape and may even cause it to pop. In the case of your eye, too much pressure can damage the optic nerve.

Fluids inside the eye help maintain the IOP. These fluids are the vitreous, which fills the vitreous cavity, at the back of the eye, and the aqueous humor, which fills the anterior chamber, at the front of the eye. Aqueous humor is continuously produced and circulated through the anterior chamber before draining out of the eye. This continuous flow of fluid nourishes the lens and the cornea and removes unwanted debris. A healthy eye produces aqueous humor at the same rate that it drains fluid, thus maintaining a normal pressure.

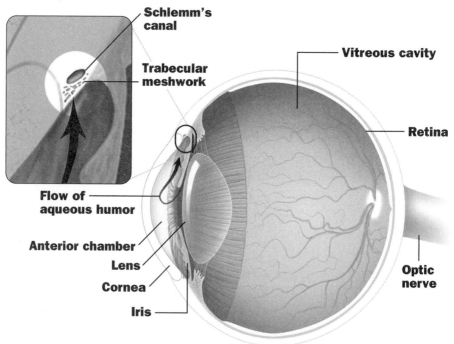

Movement of fluid in the eye
Aqueous humor continuously circulates from behind the iris into the anterior chamber. It exits the eye where the iris and the cornea meet. The fluid filters through the trabecular meshwork before passing into an open channel called Schlemm's canal.

Aqueous humor exits the eye through a drainage system located at the angle formed where the iris and the cornea meet. Here it passes through a sievelike system of spongy tissue called the trabecular meshwork and drains into a channel called Schlemm's canal. The fluid then merges into the body's bloodstream.

When the drainage system doesn't function properly — for example, if the trabecular meshwork gets clogged — the aqueous humor can't flow at its normal rate and pressure builds within the eye. For reasons not completely understood, the increased eye pressure gradually damages the nerve fibers that make up the optic nerve.

Types

There are several types of glaucoma. The differences have to do with what's causing the fluid blockage that builds pressure in the eye.

Primary open-angle

Primary open-angle glaucoma, also called chronic open-angle glaucoma, accounts for most cases of the disease. Although the drainage angle formed by the cornea and the iris remains open, the aqueous humor drains too slowly. This leads to fluid backup and a gradual

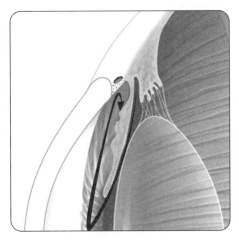

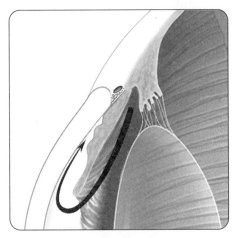

Open-angle glaucoma
Blockage of the trabecular meshwork slows drainage of the aqueous humor, which increases intraocular pressure.

Angle-closure glaucoma
The angle formed by the cornea and the iris narrows, preventing the aqueous humor from draining out of the eye. This can lead to a rapid increase in intraocular pressure.

buildup of pressure within the eye. Damage to the optic nerve is so slow and painless that a large portion of your vision can be lost before you're even aware of a problem.

The cause of primary open-angle glaucoma remains unknown. It may be that the aqueous humor drains or is absorbed less efficiently with age, but then not all older adults get this form of glaucoma.

Angle-closure

Angle-closure glaucoma, also called closed-angle glaucoma, is a less common form of the disease. It occurs when the drainage angle formed by the cornea and the iris closes or becomes blocked. The aqueous humor can't exit through the trabecular meshwork, resulting in an increase in eye pressure. Angle-closure glaucoma can be chronic (progressing gradually) or acute (coming on suddenly).

Most people with this type of glaucoma have a very narrow drainage angle, which may be an abnormality from birth. Angle-closure glaucoma is more common among farsighted people, who tend to have smaller eyes that can narrow the angle. Normal aging also may cause angle blockage. As you get older, your lens becomes larger, pushing your iris forward and narrowing the space between the iris and the cornea.

If you have a narrow drainage angle and your pupils become widely dilated, the angle may close and cause a sudden increase in eye pressure. This attack of acute angle-closure glaucoma requires immediate treatment. Although an acute attack often affects only one eye, the other eye is at risk of an attack as well.

Several factors can cause your pupils to dilate:

- Darkness or dim light
- Stress or excitement
- Certain medications, including antihistamines, tricyclic antide-pressants and eyedrops used to dilate your pupils, which may not cause the angle to close until several hours after the drops are put in

Acute angle-closure glaucoma is a medical emergency that can cause vision loss within hours of its onset. Without treatment the eye can become blind in as little as 1 or 2 days.

Secondary

Both open-angle and angle-closure glaucoma can be primary or secondary conditions. They're called primary when the cause of the condition is unknown. They're called secondary when the condition can be traced to a known cause, such as an injury or an eye disease. Secondary glaucoma may be caused by a variety of medical conditions, medications, physical injuries, and eye abnormalities or deformities. Infrequently eye surgery can cause secondary glaucoma.

Low-tension

Low-tension glaucoma is an unusual and poorly understood form of the disease. In this form, eye pressure remains within a normal range but the optic nerve is damaged nevertheless. Why this happens is unknown, although some experts believe that people with low-tension glaucoma may have an abnormally fragile optic nerve or a reduced blood supply to the optic nerve, caused by a condition such as closed arteries (atherosclerosis). Under these circumstances even normal pressure on the optic nerve is enough to cause damage.

Signs and symptoms

Primary open-angle glaucoma progresses with few or no symptoms until the condition reaches an advanced stage. As increased eye pressure continues to damage the optic nerve, you lose more and more of your peripheral vision. Open-angle glaucoma usually affects both eyes, although at first you may have symptoms in just one eye. Other symptoms include:
- Sensitivity to light and glare
- Trouble differentiating between varying shades of light and dark
- Trouble with night vision

Acute angle-closure glaucoma develops suddenly in response to a rapid rise in eye pressure. An attack often happens in the evening when the light is dim and your pupils are dilated. The symptoms may be severe. Signs and symptoms include:

- Blurred vision
- Halos around lights
- Reddening of the eye
- Headache
- Severe eye pain
- Nausea and vomiting
- Hardness of the affected eye

If you have any of these signs or symptoms, get immediate medical attention. Permanent vision loss can occur within hours of the attack.

Signs and symptoms of secondary glaucoma vary and depend on what's causing the glaucoma and whether the drainage angle is open or closed.

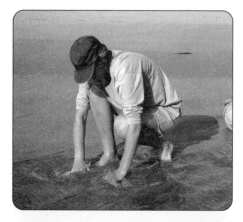

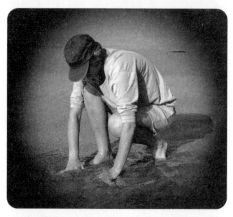

Causes

The underlying causes of glaucoma aren't completely understood. Evidence suggests that open-angle glaucoma has a genetic link. That is, a defect in one or more genes may cause the disease. People with a family history of glaucoma are more likely to develop it themselves. Nevertheless, the exact genetic defects responsible for its occurrence haven't been identified.

Other factors appear to contribute to the disease, but again,

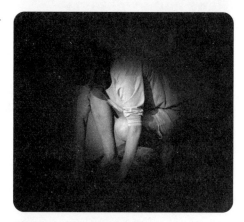

Vision with glaucoma
The gradual loss of peripheral vision is shown in this sequence from normal visual field (top) to early-stage glaucoma (center) to advanced-stage glaucoma (bottom).

what these factors are and the relationships among them aren't known for certain. Although glaucoma is normally associated with increased eye pressure, people with normal or low eye pressure can experience vision loss. And people with higher-than-normal eye pressure may never experience optic nerve damage.

Doctors have debated for many years about how damage to the optic nerve occurs. One theory holds that the pressure of backed up aqueous humor causes structural damage and ultimately death to the nerve fibers. Another theory suggests that nerve fibers die when small blood vessels that feed the optic nerve become blocked or when the blood supply is disrupted.

The cause of decreased drainage through the trabecular meshwork also presents a puzzle. The changes that slow drainage may be a result of normal aging, yet not all older adults develop glaucoma.

Risk factors

If your IOP is higher than what's considered normal, you're at increased risk of developing glaucoma. Yet most people with slightly elevated intraocular pressure don't develop the disease. This makes it difficult to predict who will get glaucoma. Certain other factors are known to increase your risk. Because chronic forms of glaucoma can destroy vision before any symptoms are apparent, it's important to be aware of these factors:

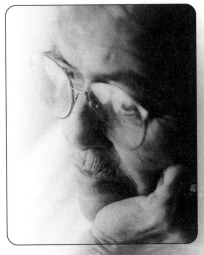

Age. Open-angle glaucoma is rare before age 40. The risk of developing glaucoma nearly doubles every 10 years after age 50. Approximately 14 percent of people in the United States who are age 80 have the disease. Primary open-angle glaucoma is most common in older adult women.

Race. In the United States, blacks are three to four times more likely to get glaucoma than are whites, and they are six times more likely to suffer permanent blindness as a result. The reasons for this difference aren't known, but blacks may be more susceptible to damage to the optic nerve, or they may not respond to current treatments as well as whites do. Asian-Americans, particularly people of Vietnamese descent, are also at higher risk. Japanese-Americans are more prone to develop low-tension glaucoma.

A family history of glaucoma. If one of your parents has glaucoma, you have about a 20 percent chance of developing the disease. If you have a sibling with the disease, your chance of getting it is about 50 percent.

Medical conditions. If you have diabetes, your risk of developing glaucoma is about three times greater than that of people who don't have diabetes. A history of high blood pressure or heart disease also can increase your risk. Other risk factors include retinal detachment, eye tumors and eye inflammations such as chronic uveitis and iritis. Previous eye surgery may trigger secondary glaucoma.

Physical injuries. Severe trauma, such as being hit in the eye, can result in increased eye pressure. Injury can also dislocate the lens, closing the drainage angle.

Nearsightedness. Severe nearsightedness increases the risk of developing glaucoma. An extensive study of eye health found that nearsighted people had a two to three times higher risk of developing glaucoma than did people who were not nearsighted.

Prolonged corticosteroid use. Using corticosteroids for prolonged periods of time puts you at risk of getting secondary glaucoma.

Eye pressure: What is normal?

Normal eye pressure ranges from 10 to 22 millimeters of mercury (mm Hg). Anyone with eye pressure over 23 mm Hg is considered at risk of developing glaucoma and needs to be carefully monitored for early signs of glaucoma. People with intraocular pressure greater than 30 mm Hg are considered at high risk.

Eye abnormalities. Structural abnormalities of the eye can lead to secondary glaucoma. For example, pigmentary glaucoma is a form of secondary glaucoma caused by pigment granules being released from the back of the iris. These granules can block the trabecular meshwork.

Screening and diagnosis

Regular eye exams are the key to detecting glaucoma early enough for successful treatment. It's best to have routine eye checkups every 2 to 4 years after age 40 and every 1 to 2 years after age 65. If you're at increased risk, your doctor may recommend more frequent monitoring. If your doctor suspects that you have glaucoma, he or she may perform a series of tests on you to detect any signs of damage.

Tests to detect glaucoma

Tonometry. Tonometry is a simple, painless procedure that measures your intraocular pressure. It is usually the initial screening test for glaucoma. Two common techniques are air-puff tonometry and applanation tonometry (see page 26). Air-puff tonometry uses a puff of air to measure the amount of force needed to indent your cornea. An applanation tonometer is a sophisticated device that's usually fitted to a slit lamp. For this extremely accurate test, your doctor numbs your eyes with drops and has you sit at the slit lamp, where a small flat-tipped cone pushes lightly against your eyeball. The force required to flatten (applanate) a small area of your cornea translates into a measure of your IOP.

Test for optic nerve damage. To check the fibers in your optic nerve, your eye doctor uses an instrument called an ophthalmoscope, which enables him or her to look directly through the pupil to the back of your eye. Your doctor may also use laser light and computers to create a three-dimensional image of your optic nerve. This can reveal slight changes that may indicate the beginnings of glaucoma.

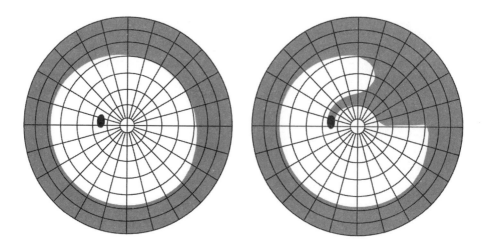

Map of visual field for the left eye showing changes from glaucoma
A normal visual field mapped by tangent screen perimetry is shown at left. The visual field map at right shows a typical pattern found in someone with glaucoma. Shading indicates that the upper-right portion of the visual field has been lost. The black spot near the center marks your blind spot (the location of the optic nerve).

Visual field test. To check how your visual field has been affected by glaucoma, the doctor uses a perimetry test. One method, known as tangent screen perimetry, requires you to look at a screen with a target in the center. Your eye doctor manipulates a small object on a wand at different locations in your visual field. You indicate whenever you see the object come into view. By repeating this process over and over again, the doctor can map your entire visual field. Another more commonly used perimetry test is described on page 25.

Other tests. To distinguish between open-angle glaucoma and angle-closure glaucoma, your eye doctor may use a technique called gonioscopy (goe-nee-OS-kuh-pee), in which a special lens is placed on the eye to inspect the drainage angle. Another test, tonography, can measure how fast fluid drains through the trabecular meshwork.

Diagnosing glaucoma
To receive a diagnosis of glaucoma, a person must exhibit several factors. These include an elevated IOP, areas of vision loss and damage to the optic nerve. In glaucoma, the optic disk will show visible

signs of damage (see figure 12 in the color section). The optic disk is the area where all the nerve fibers come together at the back of the eye before exiting the eyeball. An optic disk that has been affected by glaucoma appears indented, or excavated, as if someone scooped out part of the center of the disk. This condition is known as cupping. The normal contour and color of the disk may be affected by the loss of nerve fibers.

If your doctor determines that you have elevated IOP, an excavated optic disk and loss of visual field, you'll likely be treated for glaucoma. If you have only slightly elevated eye pressure, an undamaged optic nerve and no visual field loss, you may not need treatment but more frequent examinations may be advised to detect any future changes. If you have signs of optic nerve damage and visual field loss, even if your eye pressure is in the normal range, you may be treated to lower eye pressure further, which may help slow the progression of glaucoma.

Treatment

Glaucoma can't be cured, and damage caused by the disease can't be reversed. The good news is that with treatment, glaucoma can be controlled. Eyedrops, oral medications and surgical procedures are used to prevent or slow further damage.

If you have glaucoma, you'll need to continue treatment for the rest of your life. Because the disease can progress or change without your being aware of it, your treatment may need to be changed over time. Regular checkups and adherence to a treatment plan may seem burdensome, but they're essential to prevent vision loss.

Preventing further damage to the optic nerve and continued loss of visual field may be accomplished by keeping your eye pressure under control. Your eye doctor may focus on lowering your IOP to a level that's unlikely to cause further optic nerve damage. This level is often referred to as the target pressure and will probably be a range rather than a single number. Target pressure differs for each person, depending on the extent of the damage and other factors. Your target pressure may change over the course of your lifetime.

Eyedrops for the treatment of glaucoma

Your doctor may prescribe more than one type of eyedrop. If you're using more than one, wait 5 to 10 minutes between applications. Eyedrop types include:

Beta blockers

Function: Reduce the production of aqueous humor.

Drug names: Levobunolol (Betagan), timolol (Timoptic, Betimol), carteolol (Ocupress), betaxolol (Betoptic), metipranolol (Optipranolol).

Possible side effects: Difficulty breathing, slowed pulse, hair loss, decreased blood pressure, impotence, fatigue, weakness, depression and memory loss. If you have asthma, bronchitis or emphysema, or if you have diabetes and use insulin, beta blockers shouldn't be used unless no alternative is possible, and then only with great care.

Alpha-adrenergic agents

Function: Reduce the production of aqueous humor.

Drug names: Apraclonidine (Iopidine), brimonidine (Alphagan).

Possible side effects: Increased blood pressure, tremors, headache, anxiety, red and itchy eyes, dry mouth and allergic reactions.

Carbonic anhydrase inhibitors

Function: Reduce the amount of aqueous humor.

Drug name: Dorzolamide (Trusopt).

Possible side effects: A bad taste in the mouth. Frequent urination and a tingling sensation in the fingers and the toes are common when a carbonic anhydrase inhibitor is taken orally but rare when it is taken as drops. If you're allergic to sulfa drugs, this type of medication shouldn't be used unless no alternative is possible, and then only with great care.

Prostaglandin analogues

Function: Increase the outflow of aqueous humor. These hormonelike substances may be used in conjunction with a drug that reduces production of aqueous humor.

Drug name: Latanoprost (Xalatan).

Possible side effects: Mild reddening and stinging of the eyes and darkening of the iris and the eyelid skin.

Prostamides

Function: Increase the outflow of aqueous humor.

Drug name: Bimatoprost (Lumigan).

Possible side effects: Mild to moderate reddening of the eyes and eyelash growth.

Miotics (rarely used today)

Function: Increase the outflow of aqueous humor.

Drug names: Pilocarpine (Isopto Carpine, Pilocar, others).

Possible side effects: Pain around or inside the eyes, brow ache, blurred or dim vision, nearsightedness, allergic reactions, a stuffy nose, sweating, increased salivation and occasional digestive problems.

Epinephrine compounds (rarely used today)

Function: Increase the outflow of aqueous humor.

Drug name: Epinephrine (Epifrin, Eppy/N).

Possible side effects: Red eyes, allergic reactions, palpitations, high blood pressure, headache and anxiety.

Medications are the most common early treatment for glaucoma. Standard practice has been to move on to surgery if medications are ineffective. However, recent studies support the use of surgery as a safe and effective initial treatment.

Eyedrops
Glaucoma treatment often starts with medicated eyedrops. There are several types of drops the doctor may prescribe (see pages 94 to 95). It's important to use the drops exactly as prescribed to control your IOP. Skipping even a few doses can cause damage to the optic nerve to worsen. Some drops need to be applied several times each day, and others must be used just once a day. It's also important to inform your doctor of all medications you're currently taking, to avoid any undesirable drug interactions.

Because some of the eyedrops are absorbed into your bloodstream, you may experience side effects unrelated to your eyes. To minimize this absorption, close your eyes for 1 to 2 minutes after putting the drops in. Press lightly at the corner of your eye near your nose to close the tear duct, and wipe off any unused drops from your eyelid.

Oral medications
If eyedrops alone don't bring your eye pressure down to the desired level, your doctor may also prescribe oral medication. The most common oral medications for glaucoma are carbonic anhydrase inhibitors. These pills, which include acetazolamide (Diamox, Storzolamide, others), dichlorphenamide (Daranide) and methazolamide (Neptazane), should be taken with meals to reduce side effects. You can help to minimize the potassium loss that these medications can cause by adding bananas and apple juice to your diet.

When you first start taking these oral medications, you may experience a frequent need to urinate and a tingling sensation in the fingers and the toes. These symptoms often disappear after a few days. Other possible side effects of carbonic anhydrase inhibitors include rashes, depression, fatigue, lethargy, stomach upset, a metallic taste in carbonated beverages, impotence and weight loss. Kidney stones also can occur.

> **Treating acute angle-closure glaucoma**
>
> Acute angle-closure glaucoma is a medical emergency. When you come in with this condition, doctors may administer several medications to reduce eye pressure as quickly as possible. Once your eye pressure is under control, you'll likely have an operation called iridotomy (ir-uh-DOT-uh-mee). In this procedure the doctor uses a laser beam to create a small hole in your iris that allows aqueous humor to flow more freely into the anterior chamber. Many doctors recommend an iridotomy on the other eye at a later date because of the high risk that it too will have an attack within the next few years.

Surgery

Surgery might become necessary for the treatment of glaucoma if medications aren't effective or tolerated. Several different types of surgery are used, including laser surgery and more conventional procedures:

Laser surgery. In the last couple of decades, a procedure called trabeculoplasty (truh-BEK-yoo-loe-plas-tee) has been used increasingly in the treatment of open-angle glaucoma. The doctor uses a high energy laser beam to shrink part of the trabecular meshwork, which causes other parts of the meshwork to stretch and open up. This helps aqueous humor drain more easily from the eye.

This type of laser surgery is an office procedure that takes 10 to 20 minutes. You'll be given an anesthetic eyedrop, seated at a slit lamp and fitted with a special lens on your eye. The doctor aims the laser through the lens at the trabecular meshwork and applies burns to it. You will see bright flashes of light.

After the surgery you can immediately resume normal activities without discomfort. The doctor will check your eye pressure 1 to 2 hours after the procedure and several times in the following weeks. He or she may prescribe anti-inflammatory eyedrops for you to use for a few days following trabeculoplasty. It may take a few weeks before the full effect of the surgery becomes apparent.

In almost all cases, laser surgery for glaucoma initially lowers intraocular pressure. However, its effects may wear off over time.

Studies show that eye pressure rises in many people 2 to 5 years after they receive the laser treatment.

Conventional surgery. If eyedrops and laser surgery aren't effective in controlling your eye pressure, you may need an operation called a trabeculectomy (truh-bek-yoo-LEK-tuh-mee). This procedure is done in a hospital or an outpatient surgery center. You'll receive medication to help you relax and eyedrops and an injection of anesthetic to numb your eye. Using delicate instruments under an operating microscope, the surgeon creates an opening in the sclera and removes a small piece of the trabecular meshwork. The aqueous humor can now freely leave the eye through this hole. As a result your eye pressure will be lowered The hole is covered by the conjunctiva, so there's not an open hole in your eye.

Your doctor will check your eye in several follow-up visits. You'll use antibiotic and anti-inflammatory eyedrops for some time after the operation to fight infection and scarring of the newly created drainage opening. Scarring is a particular problem for young adults, blacks and people who have had cataract surgery. This procedure works best if you haven't had any previous eye surgery.

Although glaucoma surgery may preserve current vision, it can't restore already lost vision. Sometimes a single surgical procedure may not lower eye pressure enough, in which case you'll need to continue using glaucoma drops or have another trabeculectomy operation.

Drainage implants. Another type of operation, called drainage implant surgery, may be performed on people with secondary glaucoma or children with glaucoma.

Like the trabeculectomy, drainage implant surgery is performed at a hospital or an outpatient clinic. You'll be given medication to help you relax and eyedrops and anesthetic to numb the eye. Then the doctor inserts a small silicone tube in your eye to help drain aqueous humor.

After the surgery you'll wear an eye patch for 24 hours and use eyedrops for several weeks to fight infection and scarring. Your doctor will check your eyes several times in the weeks that follow.

Complications from glaucoma surgery may include infection,

bleeding, eye pressure that remains too high or too low and, potentially, loss of vision. Having eye surgery may also speed up the development of cataracts. Most of these complications can be effectively treated.

Self-care

The best way to prevent damage from glaucoma is to know your risk factors and have regular eye exams. If you have glaucoma, the most important thing you can do is take your medications exactly as prescribed. Frequent eye exams will help your doctor monitor your eye pressure and keep you and your doctor aware of any changes in your vision.

Here are other self-care tips:

Maintain a healthy diet. Vitamins and minerals that are important for the eyes include vitamin A, vitamin C, vitamin E, zinc and copper. Drink fluids in small amounts over the course of a day. Drinking a quart or more of any liquid within a short time may increase eye pressure. Limit caffeine to low or moderate levels.

Get regular exercise. Studies show that people with open-angle glaucoma who exercise regularly — at least three times a week — can reduce their eye pressure by an average of 20 percent. However, angle-closure glaucoma isn't affected by exercise, and people with pigmentary glaucoma, a form of secondary glaucoma, may experience increased eye pressure after exercise. Talk to your doctor about an appropriate exercise program.

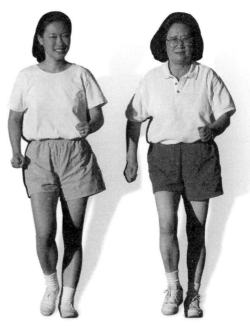

Steer clear of herbal remedies. A number of herbal supplements, such as bilberry, are advertised as glaucoma remedies. Bilberry is not effective in preventing or treating glaucoma. Be cautious about herbal supplements, and discuss them with your doctor before trying them.

Find healthy ways to cope with stress. Stress can trigger an attack of acute angle-closure glaucoma. Relaxation techniques, such as meditation and progressive muscle relaxation, may be helpful in dealing with stress.

Wear sunglasses with full ultraviolet protection. Whenever you're out in the sun, even if only for a few minutes, wear sunglasses that block ultraviolet (UV) light.

Wear proper eye protection. Eye trauma can result in increased eye pressure. Use safety glasses or goggles when you play sports, use tools or machinery, or work with chemicals.

Chapter 7

Cataracts

A cataract is a clouding of the normally clear lens of the eye. The Latin word *cataracta* means "waterfall" — imagine trying to peer through a sheet of falling water or through a frosty or fogged-up window. Clouded vision can make it more difficult to read, drive a car or see the expression on a friend's face. Cataracts commonly affect distance vision and cause problems with glare. They generally do not cause pain, double vision with both eyes or abnormal tearing.

The most common type of cataract is related to aging. Clouding of the lens is a normal part of getting older, sort of like gray hair or wrinkles. Almost all Americans age 65 and older have some degree of clouding of the lens. Most cataracts develop slowly and don't disturb your eyesight early on. But as the clouding progresses, it eventually interferes with your clear vision.

The key to living with cataracts is knowing when it's time not to live with them anymore. In the early stages, stronger lighting and eyeglasses can help you deal with the vision problems. But at a certain point, if your normal lifestyle is jeopardized by impaired vision, you might need surgery. Thanks to enormous advances in the management of this condition, cataract removal is one of the safest, most effective and most common surgical procedures — one that restores the sight of millions of Americans.

Cataract myths

Perhaps because cataracts are one of the most common eye disorders, many misconceptions about them exist. Here are the
facts:

- A cataract is not a film covering your eye. It's located within the eye — in the lens.
- Just because your eye looks clear doesn't mean there's no
  cataract. Most cataracts are detectable only with special
  instruments.
- Cataracts aren't caused by cancer.
- Cataracts don't spread from one eye to the other, although
  both eyes may be affected.
- Overusing your eyes doesn't cause cataracts.
- You don't have to wait for a cataract to turn completely
  white or become "ripe" before having it removed.

Types

A cataract can develop in one or both eyes, and it may or may not
affect the entire lens (see figure 11 in the color section). The lens is
located just behind the iris and the pupil. It's shaped like a magnifying glass — thick in the middle and thinner near the edges. Tiny
ligaments, which are bands of tough tissue fiber, hold it in place.

When your eyes work properly, light passes through the cornea
and the pupil to the lens. The lens focuses this light, producing
clear, sharp images on the retina, the light-sensitive membrane on
the back inside wall of your eyeball that functions like the film of
a camera. The clouding of the lens, or cataract, scatters the light
and prevents a sharply defined image from reaching the retina.
Your vision becomes blurred.

The lens consists of three layers. The outer layer is a thin, clear
membrane called the capsule. It surrounds a soft, clear material
called the cortex. The hard center of the lens is the nucleus. If you
think of the lens as a piece of fruit, the capsule is the skin, the cortex is the fleshy fruit, and the nucleus is the pit. A cataract can
form in any part of the lens.

Nuclear

A nuclear cataract is the most common type of cataract and the one most associated with aging. It occurs in the center of the lens. In its early stages, as the lens changes the way it focuses light, you may become more nearsighted or experience a temporary improvement in your reading vision. Some people actually stop needing their glasses. Unfortunately, this so-called second sight disappears as the lens gradually turns yellow or greenish and begins to cloud vision. As the cataract progresses, the lens may even turn brown. You may have particular problems seeing in dim light and find driving at night especially troublesome.

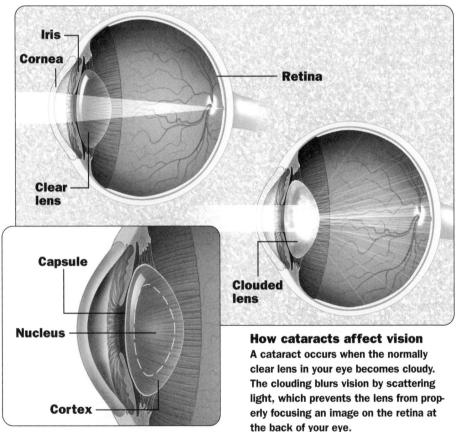

Parts of the lens
For many people a cataract develops as a normal part of aging. It can form in any one of the layers of the lens — the nucleus, the cortex or the capsule.

How cataracts affect vision
A cataract occurs when the normally clear lens in your eye becomes cloudy. The clouding blurs vision by scattering light, which prevents the lens from properly focusing an image on the retina at the back of your eye.

Cortical

A cortical cataract begins as whitish, wedge-shaped streaks on the outer edge of the lens cortex. As it slowly progresses, the streaks extend to the center and interfere with light passing through the nucleus. Both your distance and near vision can be significantly impaired. Focusing problems and distortion are common. You may also have problems with glare and loss of contrast. Many people with diabetes develop cortical cataracts. Cortical cataracts are the only type of cataract associated with exposure to ultraviolet (UV) light.

Subcapsular

A subcapsular cataract starts as a small, opaque area just under the capsule shell. It usually forms at the back of the lens, right in the path of light on its way to the retina. This type of cataract may occur in both eyes but will tend to be more advanced in one eye than the other. A subcapsular cataract often interferes with your reading vision, reduces your vision in bright light and causes glare or halos around lights at night. You're more likely to develop a subcapsular cataract if you have diabetes, are very nearsighted, have taken corticosteroid drugs or have had an eye injury or eye surgery.

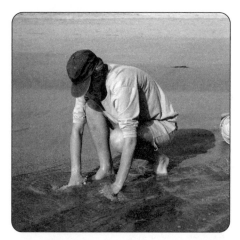 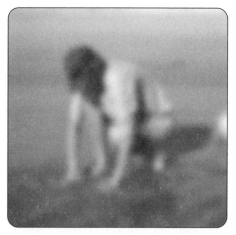

Vision with cataracts
Normal vision (left) becomes blurred as a cataract forms (right).

Signs and symptoms

A cataract usually develops slowly and causes no pain. At first the cloudiness may affect only a small part of the lens, and you may be unaware of any vision loss. Over time, however, as the cataract grows larger, it clouds more of the lens. When significantly less light reaches the retina, your vision becomes impaired.

Symptoms of a cataract include:
- Clouded, blurred or dim vision
- Increasing difficulty with vision at night
- Sensitivity to light and glare
- Halos around lights
- The need for brighter light for reading and other activities
- Frequent changes in eyeglass or contact lens prescriptions
- The fading or yellowing of colors
- Double vision or multiple vision in one eye

If you have a cataract, light from the sun, lamps or oncoming headlights may seem too bright. Glare and halos around lights can make driving uncomfortable and dangerous. You may experience eyestrain or find yourself blinking more often to clear your vision.

Keep in mind that cataracts don't typically cause any change in the appearance of the eye or the production of tears. Pain, redness, itching, irritation, aching in the eye or a discharge from the eye may be signs and symptoms of other eye disorders.

A cataract isn't dangerous to the physical health of your eye unless the cataract becomes completely white, a condition known as an overripe (hypermature) cataract. This can cause inflammation, pain and headache. A hypermature cataract is extremely rare but needs to be removed quickly.

Causes

As you age the lenses in your eyes become less flexible, less transparent and thicker. The lens is made mostly of water and protein fibers. The protein fibers are arranged in a precise manner that makes the lens clear and allows light to pass through without interference. With aging, the composition of the lens undergoes changes and the structure of the protein fibers breaks down. Some of the fibers begin to clump together, clouding small areas of the lens. As the cataract continues to develop, the clouding becomes more dense and involves a greater part of the lens.

Scientists don't know why a lens changes with age. One possibility is damage caused by unstable molecules known as free radicals. Smoking and exposure to UV light are two sources of free radicals. General wear and tear on the lens over the years also may cause the changes in protein fibers.

Age-related changes in the lens aren't the only cause of cataracts. Some people are born with cataracts or develop them in childhood. Such cataracts may be the result of the mother having contracted rubella (German measles) during pregnancy. They may also be due to a chemical imbalance or developmental problem. Congenital cataracts, as they're called, don't always affect vision, but if they do they're usually removed soon after detection.

Risk factors

Everyone is at risk of developing cataracts simply because age is the single greatest risk factor. And everyone by age 65 has some degree of lens clouding, although it may not impair vision. Cataracts are more common in women than in men, and they're more common in blacks than in whites.

Other factors that increase your risk of cataracts include:
- Diabetes
- A family history of cataracts
- Previous eye injury or inflammation
- Previous eye surgery
- Prolonged corticosteroid use
- Excessive consumption of alcohol
- Excessive exposure to sunlight
- Exposure to high levels of radiation, such as from cancer therapy
- Smoking

Screening and diagnosis

The only way to know for sure if you have a cataract is to have an eye examination that includes a visual acuity test, a slit-lamp examination and a retinal exam (ophthalmoscopy). The eye doctor will dilate your pupil to examine the lens for signs of a cataract and, if needed, determine how dense the clouding is. He or she will also check for glaucoma and, if you have blurred vision or discomfort, for other problems with the retina and the optic nerve. If you have a cataract, you can discuss treatment options with your eye doctor. If in addition to having a cataract you have severe glaucoma or another serious eye condition, removing the cataract may not result in improved vision.

Treatment

The only effective treatment for a cataract is surgery to remove the clouded lens and replace it with a clear lens implant. Cataracts can't be cured with medications, dietary supplements, exercise or optical devices.

In the early stages of a cataract, when symptoms are mild, a good understanding of the condition and a willingness to adjust your lifestyle can help. You can try a few simple approaches to deal with symptoms:

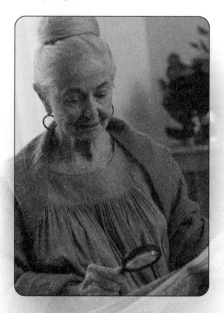

- If you have eyeglasses or contact lenses, make sure they're the most accurate prescription possible.
- Use a magnifying glass to read.
- Improve the lighting in your home with more or brighter lamps, for example, those that can accommodate halo-

An eye on history

Years ago having a cataract removed was an ordeal involving several days in the hospital, painful stitches in the eye and a recovery spent lying on your back with your head held in place with sandbags. Afterward you had to wear thick "Coke-bottle" eyeglasses. Luckily things have changed dramatically.

Modern surgical treatment of cataracts started with the development of the intraocular lens in 1949 by Dr. Harold Ridley, an English ophthalmologist. Dr. Ridley recalled the experience of eye doctors who had treated Royal Air Force pilots during World War II. Some pilots had bits of hard plastic lodged in their eye after their plane's cockpit shattered. To the doctors' surprise, these fragments didn't cause any serious problems in the pilots' eyes. With this in mind, Ridley began experimenting with making artificial lenses from plastic.

Phacoemulsification was developed in the mid-1960s by American ophthalmologist Dr. Charles Kelman. Since then advances in surgical techniques and lens replacement have made cataract surgery one of the safest and most effective surgeries. The number of cataract surgeries done each year has increased phenomenally in the United States and Europe.

And what does the future hold? One area of research is the use of lasers in phacoemulsification. Other surgical techniques are being investigated, and researchers are also looking at ways to prevent cataract formation with drugs.

gen lights or 100- to 150-watt incandescent bulbs. When you go outside during the day, wear sunglasses to reduce glare.

• Limit your night driving.

These measures may help for a while, but as the cataract progresses, your vision may deteriorate futher. When vision loss starts to interfere with your everyday activities, you'll want to consider cataract surgery.

Cataract surgery is the most common surgery performed on Americans age 65 and older. More than 1.5 million cataract operations are performed each year. And this surgery is very successful in restoring vision — more than 95 percent of people who have a cataract removed end up with better vision. Many people report not only better vision but a reduction in the power of their lens prescription and improvements in the overall quality of their life after the operation.

When is the right time to have a cataract removed?
The decision to have cataract surgery is one that you and your eye doctor will make together. You'll probably have plenty of time to consider and discuss your options carefully. In most cases waiting until you're ready to have surgery won't harm your eye. You may not need cataract surgery for many years if at all. In younger people or those with diabetes, however, cataracts may develop more quickly.

Base your decision on your degree of vision loss and your ability to function in daily life. In general, surgery is recommended if the results of your visual acuity test are 20/50 or worse, even with eyeglasses, but this figure isn't set in stone. Think about how the cataract affects your daily life. Can you see to do your job or drive safely? Can you read or watch television in comfort? Is it difficult to cook, shop, do yardwork, climb stairs or take medications? How active are you? Does lack of vision affect your level of independence? Are you afraid you'll trip or fall or bump into something?

The answers to these questions are different for each person. An older person who isn't very active may have less need for sharp vision than a younger person who needs to drive a car and earn a living. Some people with only minor vision loss from a cataract might want surgery because of problems with glare or double vision. Sometimes a cataract should be removed even if it doesn't cause major problems with vision, for example, if it's preventing the treatment of another eye problem, such as age-related macular degeneration, diabetic retinopathy or retinal detachment.

If you have cataracts in both eyes and decide to have surgery, your ophthalmologist typically removes the cataract in one eye at a time. This allows time for the first eye to heal before the second eye is operated on.

Vision and lens implants

Most lens implants, or intraocular lenses (IOLs), are monofocal, that is, they have a fixed point of focus and are suitable for either near vision or distance vision but not both. If a distance lens is implanted, you will need to wear glasses or contact lenses for reading; if a reading lens is implanted, you will need glasses for seeing far away. Most monofocal implants correct for distance vision.

In 1997 the Food and Drug Administration approved the first multifocal lens. In theory these lenses correct near vision and distance vision simultaneously. Because they are a compromise, with these IOLs your near vision and distance vision will improve but not as much as, for example, your distance vision alone would have improved if you had received a monofocal IOL corrected for distance. With multifocal IOLs you may experience problems with glare, halos, loss of contrast and night driving. In addition, multifocal IOLs need to be implanted in both eyes.

A recent study found that many people could stop wearing eyeglasses or contact lenses after receiving multifocal implants. For now the multifocal lens still has some glare problems that need to be worked out. Researchers continue to try to resolve these problems and improve IOLs so that they are flexible enough for the eye to focus at both distant and near objects.

What happens during cataract surgery?

Important advances in surgical technique and more sophisticated technology have helped make surgery a safe and effective treatment for cataracts. Two things happen during cataract surgery — the clouded lens is removed, and a clear artificial lens is inserted.

Prior to surgery, your eye doctor will measure the size and shape of your eye to determine the proper lens implant power. This measurement is made with a painless ultrasound test. Cataract surgery is typically an outpatient procedure that takes less than an hour. Most people are awake, relaxed and comfortable during the surgery, needing only local anesthesia. On rare occasions some people may need to be put under general anesthesia.

Removing the cataract. The most commonly used proce
to remove a cataract is called phacoemulsification (fak-o-e-n
sih-fih-KA-shun), in which the surgeon removes the cataract
while leaving most of the lens capsule (outer layer) in place.
The capsule will help support the lens implant when it's
inserted. An alternative procedure called extracapsular cataract
extraction is similar to phacoemulsification but requires a
larger incision.

Phacoemulsification. During phacoemulsification, phaco for
short, the surgeon makes a small incision, about 1/8 inch (3 mm),
where the cornea meets the conjunctiva and inserts a needle-thin
probe. The surgeon then uses the probe, which vibrates with ultrasound waves, to break up (emulsify) the cataract and suction out
the fragments. The lens capsule is left in place to provide support
for the lens implant.

Extracapsular cataract extraction. If your cataract has advanced
beyond the point where phacoemulsification can effectively break
up the clouded lens, the surgeon may do an extracapsular cataract
extraction. This procedure requires a larger incision, about 3/8 inch
(10 mm), where the cornea and conjunctiva meet. Through this
opening the surgeon opens the lens capsule, removes the nucleus in
one piece and vacuums out the softer lens cortex, leaving the capsule shell in place.

Implanting the lens. Once the cataract has been removed
through phacoemulsification or the extracapsular method, a clear
artificial lens is implanted into the empty lens capsule to replace
the original clouded lens. This lens implant, also known as an
intraocular lens (IOL), is made of plastic, acrylic or silicone. It
requires no care and becomes a permanent part of your eye.
Whether or not you wore glasses before surgery, after surgery
you'll likely need reading glasses.

Some IOLs are rigid plastic and implanted through an incision
that requires several stitches (sutures) to close. However, many
IOLs are flexible, allowing a smaller incision that requires no stitches. The surgeon can fold this type of lens and insert it into the
empty capsule where the natural lens used to be. Once in place the
lens unfolds to about 1/4 inch (6 mm).

The second cataract

You may have heard of a second cataract, or "aftercataract."
This condition occurs when the back of the lens capsule — the
part of the lens that wasn't removed during surgery and that
now supports the lens implant — eventually becomes cloudy
and blurs your vision. Another term for this condition is posteri-
or capsule opacification (PCO). PCO can develop months or
years after cataract surgery. It happens about 15 percent to 20
percent of the time. The gradual clouding is the result of cell
growth on the back of the capsule.

Treatment for PCO is simple and quick. It involves a technique called YAG laser capsulotomy, in which a laser beam is
used to make a small opening in the clouded capsule to let light
pass through. *Capsulotomy* means "cutting into the capsule," and
YAG is an abbreviation of yttrium-aluminum-garnet, the type of
laser used for the procedure.

Laser capsulotomy is a painless outpatient procedure that
usually takes less than 5 minutes. After the procedure you typically stay in the doctor's office for about an hour to make sure
your eye pressure isn't elevated. In some people, particularly
those who have glaucoma or are extremely nearsighted, YAG
laser surgery can raise eye pressure. Other complications are rare
but can include swelling of the macula and a detached retina.

After cataract surgery

With phacoemulsification and foldable lens implants, surgical inci-
sions are very small, and no sutures are required. If all goes well
you'll heal fast, and your vision will start to improve within a few
days. If your surgery required a larger incision and sutures, full
healing might take about 4 weeks.

Normally you can go home on the same day as surgery, but you
won't be able to drive, so make sure to arrange for a ride home.
You'll typically see your eye doctor the next day and during the
next 4 to 6 weeks so that he or she can check the healing progress.

It's normal to feel mild discomfort for a couple of days after
surgery. Avoid rubbing or pressing on your eye. Clean your eyelids

with tissue or cotton balls to remove any crusty discharge. You may wear an eye patch or protective shield the day of surgery. Your doctor may prescribe medications to prevent infection and control eye pressure. After a couple of days, all discomfort should disappear.

Contact your doctor immediately if you experience any of the following signs or symptoms after cataract surgery. You may have developed a rare but very serious infection known as endophthalmitis (en-dof-thul-MI-tis).

- Vision loss
- Pain that persists despite the use of over-the-counter pain medications
- A significant increase in eye redness
- Light flashes or multiple spots (floaters) in front of your eye
- Nausea, vomiting or excessive coughing

Most people will need to wear glasses after cataract surgery. Astigmatism (see pages 13 to 14) is common but is less of a problem when the surgery involves a small incision. You can usually get a final prescription for eyeglasses 3 to 6 weeks after surgery.

Complications after cataract surgery are relatively rare, and most can be treated. They include inflammation, infection, bleeding, swelling, retinal detachment and glaucoma. The risks are greater for people who have other eye diseases or serious medical problems. Occasionally cataract surgery fails to improve vision because of conditions such as glaucoma or macular degeneration. It is important to evaluate and treat these other eye problems, if possible, before making the decision to proceed with cataract surgery.

Can cataracts be prevented?

Most cataracts occur with age and can't be avoided altogether. Regular eye exams remain the key to their early detection. You can take steps to help slow or prevent the development of cataracts:

- Don't smoke. Smoking produces free radicals, increasing your risk of cataracts.
- Eat a balanced diet with plenty of fruits and vegetables. For tips on a healthy diet, see pages 62 to 64.

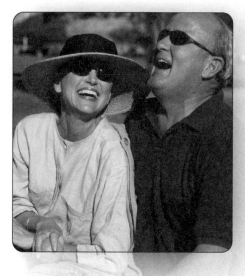

- Limit alcohol. Excessive drinking may increase your risk of developing cataracts.
- Protect yourself from the sun. Ultraviolet light may contribute to the devlopment of cataracts. It's good to wear sunglasses when you are outdoors. For tips on sun safety, see page 57.
- Follow your treatment plan if you have diabetes or other medical conditions.

Researchers continue to explore new ways to prevent and treat cataracts. If you do have a cataract, your chances of fully restoring your vision with cataract surgery are excellent if you have no other eye diseases.

Chapter 8

Diabetic retinopathy

Diabetes affects your body from head to toe. That includes your eyes. The most common and most serious eye complication of diabetes is diabetic retinopathy. *Retinopathy* is the medical term for damage to the many capillaries (tiny blood vessels) that nourish the retina. These blood vessels are often affected by the high blood sugar levels associated with diabetes.

The longer you have diabetes, the more likely it is you'll develop diabetic retinopathy. After having type 1 diabetes (formerly called juvenile or insulin-dependent diabetes) for 20 years, almost everyone with this condition has some degree of retinopathy. After the same number of years, more than 60 percent of people with type 2 diabetes (formerly called adult-onset or noninsulin-dependent diabetes) have some degree of retinopathy. Initially, most people with diabetic retinopathy experience only mild vision problems. But the condition can worsen and threaten your vision. Diabetic retinopathy is the leading cause of legal blindness among adults in the United States.

The threat of blindness is scary. But there's more cause for hope than for alarm. With early detection and treatment, the risk of severe vision loss from diabetic retinopathy is less than 5 percent. And you can take steps to protect your sight if you have diabetes. Start with a yearly eye examination. Work to keep your blood sugar and blood pressure under the best possible control.

Types

There are two types of diabetic retinopathy. Usually both eyes are affected, although the disease may be more advanced in one eye than the other.

Nonproliferative diabetic retinopathy

Nonproliferative diabetic retinopathy (NPDR), also called background diabetic retinopathy, is an early stage of the disease. It's the most common type of retinopathy, and symptoms are often mild.

In NPDR the walls of blood vessels in the retina weaken. Tiny bulges called microaneurysms (MY-kroe-an-yuh-riz-umz) protrude from the vessel walls. Another term for this is *outpouching*. The microaneurysms may begin to leak, oozing fluid and blood into the retina. As NPDR progresses, other signs of damage appear. These include patches of swollen nerve fibers, which are called cotton wool spots because they look like fluffy wisps of cotton.

Mild NPDR may not affect your ability to see clearly. Vision problems from more severe NPDR are usually the result of swelling of the macula (macular edema) or the closing of capillaries, which reduces blood flow to the macula (macular ischemia). When the macula can't function properly, your central vision decreases. Your peripheral vision usually remains normal.

Proliferative diabetic retinopathy

Proliferative diabetic retinopathy (PDR) is the more advanced form of this disease. About half the people with very severe NPDR progress to PDR within 1 year. Retinopathy becomes proliferative when abnormal new blood vessels grow (proliferate) on the retina or the optic nerve. The blood vessels also grow into the vitreous, the clear, jellylike substance that fills the center of the eye.

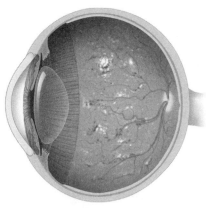

Nonproliferative diabetic retinopathy
Microanerysms, hemorrhages and cotton wool spots may often be seen in the retina.

This abnormal growth follows the widespread closing of capillaries in the retina due to high blood sugar levels. The condition can cause vision loss affecting both your central and peripheral vision. The new blood vessels may leak blood into the vitreous, which clouds or even blocks your vision. Other complications include detachment of the retina due to scar tissue formation and a form of glaucoma associated with the growth of abnormal blood vessels on the iris.

Signs and symptoms

In the early, most treatable stages of diabetic retinopathy, you usually experience no visual symptoms or pain. The disease can even progress to an advanced stage without any noticeable change in your vision.

Symptoms of diabetic retinopathy can include:

- "Spiders," "cobwebs" or tiny specks floating in your vision
- Dark streaks or a red film that blocks vision
- Vision loss, usually in both eyes, but more so in one eye than the other
- Blurred vision that may fluctuate
- A dark or empty spot in the center of your vision
- Poor night vision
- Difficulty adjusting from bright light to dim light

Causes

If you have diabetes, your body doesn't produce or use sugar (glucose) properly. Sugar in the blood is vital to your health because it's the main source of energy for your body's cells. But too much sugar in the blood can cause a host of problems. For one thing it damages the capillaries that supply nutrients to organs and tissues such as the brain, the nerves, the kidneys and the eyes.

Damage to the retina from high blood sugar occurs when microaneurysms form on the walls of the small blood vessels. The

Blurred vision in diabetes

Blurred vision is commonly brought on by fluctuations in blood sugar. Prolonged periods of excessive blood sugar cause sugar and its breakdown products to accumulate in the lens. This accumulation sucks up water and makes the lens swell, resulting in nearsightedness — meaning distant objects appear blurry to you. The nearsightedness subsides once your blood sugar is brought under steady control.

Blurred vision can also be caused by macular edema or swelling, regardless of your blood sugar level. This is cause for greater concern because macular edema often develops in people with diabetic retinopathy. The swelling may fluctuate during the day, making your vision get better or worse. If blood vessels in your eye are hemorrhaging, you might notice spots floating in your field of vision temporarily. These small spots are often followed within a few days or weeks by larger spots or clouds, which are caused by more massive hemorrhaging.

vessel walls become porous, leaking fluid into the retina (see figures 17 and 18 in the color section). Extensive leakage can leave deposits of fatty material in the retina. When swelling happens in the macula, vision may be reduced or blurred.

As vessel walls weaken, the blood vessels may close off, reducing blood flow and depriving the retina of oxygen. This can trigger proliferative diabetic retinopathy, when the oxygen-starved retina grows new blood vessels. Unfortunately, these new blood vessels don't resupply the retina with a normal blood flow. Instead they may produce other complications:

Vitreous hemorrhage. The new blood vessels may bleed (hemorrhage) into the vitreous (see figure 19 in the color section). If the amount of bleeding is small, you might see only a few dark spots or floaters. In more severe cases, blood can completely fill the vitreous cavity and block all of your vision. Vitreous hemorrhage by itself usually doesn't cause permanent vision loss. The blood eventually clears from the eye — usually within a few months — and your vision returns to its previous clarity, unless the retina is damaged.

Traction retinal detachment. The new blood vessels are often accompanied by the growth of scar tissue. The scar tissue eventually shrinks. As it shrinks it pulls the retina away from the back wall of the eye. This causes blank or blurred areas in your field of vision.

Neovascular glaucoma. The proliferation of blood vessels on the retina may be accompanied by the growth of abnormal new blood vessels on the iris. This can interfere with the normal flow of fluid out of the eye and cause pressure in the eye to build up. The result is neovascular glaucoma, a serious complication of diabetic retinopathy that can cause pain, vision loss and, if not treated successfully, the loss of the eye.

Risk factors

People with diabetes are at risk of retinopathy, whether they have type 1 or type 2 diabetes. Their risk increases the longer they have the disease. This puts people with type 1 diabetes at especially high risk because they usually become diabetic at a young age. If you were over 30 when you first got diabetes, your risk is lower, but for some people in this group, retinopathy may be the first sign of diabetes. Whatever your age, if you need to take insulin, your risk of retinopathy is higher.

Other risk factors for diabetic retinopathy include:

- Poorly controlled blood sugar levels.
- Kidney disease.
- High blood pressure.
- High blood fats (elevated levels of low-density lipoprotein cholesterol and triglycerides).
- Pregnancy. Women with type 1 diabetes who become pregnant have about a 10 percent risk of developing NPDR. Women who already have NPDR when they become pregnant tend to experience a progression of the disease, although it may improve after delivery. Less than 10 percent of pregnant women with mild NPDR develop PDR.
- Obesity.
- Infections.

Diagnosis

A common misconception among people with diabetes is, "If I can see well, there's nothing wrong with my eyes." That's false confidence. The majority of people who lose their sight because of diabetic retinopathy do so because they didn't seek early medical attention. It bears repeating: If you have diabetes, you *are* at risk even if you don't have any apparent vision problems. For this reason regular eye examinations are essential.

When and how often do you need your eyes checked? The American Academy of Ophthalmology recommends the following schedule:

- People who receive a diagnosis of diabetes before age 30 should have a comprehensive eye exam by the time diabetes has been present for 5 years or when the person is 10 years old, whichever is later.
- People who receive a diagnosis at age 30 or older should have a baseline eye exam at the time of the diagnosis.
- Women with diabetes who are pregnant or intending to become pregnant should have an eye exam before conception or early in the first trimester and thereafter every 3 months.

After the initial exam, people with diabetes should have their eyes checked every year, unless they have eye conditions that require more frequent monitoring.

See your eye doctor promptly if your eyes become painful and red, your vision decreases, or you see floaters or light flashes. If diabetic retinopathy is found, the course of treatment will depend on the severity of the condition and whether your vision is currently impaired or threatened by the retinal changes.

Treatment

If you have mild NPDR, you may not require treatment right away. However, your eye doctor will need to closely monitor your retina. More advanced forms of retinopathy often require prompt surgical treatment. The two main treatments for diabetic retinopathy are

Diagnosing retinopathy

Your eye doctor will likely diagnose diabetic retinopathy, either nonproliferative or proliferative, if the eye examination reveals any of the following:

- Leaking blood vessels
- Microaneurysms
- A swollen retina
- Fatty deposits (exudates) on the retina
- Cotton wool spots (areas of nerve fiber damage)
- Changes in blood vessels (closures, beading, loops)
- Formation of new blood vessels (neovascularization)
- Retinal hemorrhage
- Vitreous hemorrhage
- Scar tissue formation with retinal detachment

photocoagulation and vitrectomy. In a majority of cases, these treatments are effective and slow or stop the progression of the disease for some time. But they're not a cure. Because diabetes continues to affect your body, you may experience further retinal damage and vision loss at a later time.

Photocoagulation

The goal of photocoagulation is to stop the leakage of blood and fluid in the retina and thus slow the progression of diabetic retinopathy. The decision to use the procedure will depend on the type of diabetic retinopathy you have, its severity and how well it may respond to treatment.

Photocoagulation may be recommended if you have:

- Macular edema, a swelling that involves or threatens the center of the retina
- Severe NPDR, especially if you have type 2 diabetes
- PDR
- Neovascular glaucoma

In photocoagulation a high energy laser beam creates small burns in areas of the retina with abnormal blood vessel to seal any leaks. The procedure takes place in a doctor's office or an outpa-

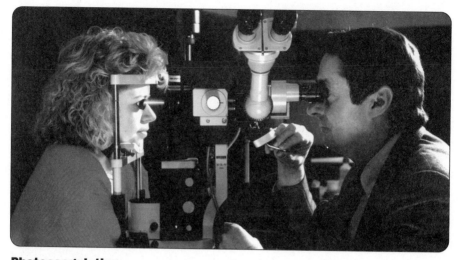

Photocoagulation
A special lens placed on the eye (left) focuses laser light onto areas of the retina where there is leakage of blood, swelling or growth of abnormal blood vessels.

tient surgical center. Before surgery your eye doctor will dilate your pupil and apply anesthetic drops to numb your eye. In some cases he or she will numb the eye more completely by injecting anesthetic around and behind the eye.

With your chin and forehead resting in a slit lamp, a medical contact lens is placed on your cornea to help focus laser light onto the sections of the retina to be treated. Fluorescein angiographic photographs (see page 29) may serve as maps to show where the laser burns should be placed. During the procedure you may see bright flashes from the short bursts of high energy light.

To treat macular edema, the laser is focused on spots where blood vessels are leaking near the macula. The doctor makes "spot welds" to stop the leakage. If the leaks are small, the laser is applied directly to specific points where the leaks occur (focal laser treatment). If the leakage is widespread, laser burns are applied in a grid pattern over a broad area (grid laser treatment).

Shortly after laser treatment, you can usually return home, but you won't be able to drive, so make sure to arrange for a ride. Your vision will be blurry for about a day. You may have some eye pain or a headache and be sensitive to light. An eye patch and over-the-counter pain relievers should help to ease the discomfort.

Even when laser surgery is successful in sealing the leaks, new areas of leakage may appear later. For this reason you'll have follow-up visits and, if necessary, additional laser treatments.

Immediately following laser surgery to treat macular edema, small spots caused by the laser burns may appear in your visual field. The spots generally fade and disappear with time. If you had blurred vision from macular edema before surgery, you may not recover completely normal vision.

Vitrectomy

Often a vitreous hemorrhage will clear up on its own. But photocoagulation treatment will be impossible if the hemorrhage is massive and doesn't clear. That's when a vitrectomy becomes necessary to restore sight or prevent total loss of vision. Early vitrectomy is especially beneficial for people with complications of type 1 diabetes.

In this procedure the surgeon uses delicate instruments to remove the blood-filled vitreous. A vitreous cutter cuts the tissue and removes it, piece by piece, from the eye. An infusion cannula,

---

Panretinal photocoagulation

For proliferative diabetic retinopathy, a form of laser surgery called panretinal or scatter photocoagulation is used. With this technique the entire retina except the macula is treated with randomly placed laser burns. The treatment causes the abnormal new blood vessels to shrink and disappear. Thus it reduces the chances of vitreous hemorrhage. Panretinal photocoagulation is usually done in two or more sessions. The treatment significantly reduces the risk of severe vision loss.

If the treatment is extensive, you may notice some loss of peripheral vision afterward. Panretinal photocoagulation is a trade-off. Some of your side vision is sacrificed to save as much of your central vision as possible. You may also notice more difficulties with your night vision and temporary blurring of your central vision. Panretinal photocoagulation doesn't always stop loss of vision from diabetic retinopathy, even with repeated treatments.

or tube, replaces the volume of removed tissue with a balanced salt solution to maintain the normal shape and pressure of the eye. A light probe illuminates the inside of the eye. The surgeon performs the procedure while looking through a microscope suspended over the eye. In this way the vitreous blood is removed to re-establish clear vision.

A vitrectomy is also used to remove scar tissue when it begins to pull the retina away from the wall of the eye. This allows a detached retina to settle back and flatten out. Your eye doctor may decide not to operate on a retina detached by scar tissue if the detachment is located away from the macula and doesn't appear to be progressing.

During a vitrectomy the surgeon may also perform panretinal photocoagulation with a laser probe. This can prevent renewed growth of abnormal blood vessels and bleeding.

Vitrectomy is usually done under local anesthesia on an outpatient basis. Your eye will be red, swollen and sensitive to light for some

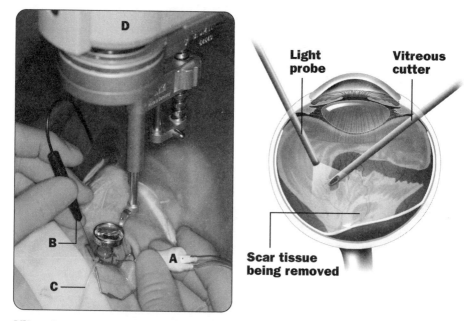

Vitrectomy

The external view (left) shows three instruments inserted into the eyeball: a vitreous cutter to remove tissue (A), a light probe for illumination (B) and an infusion cannula to replace removed tissue with fluid (C). The surgeon views the inside of the eye through a surgical microscope (D). The internal view (right) shows the cutter removing scar tissue and the light probe illuminating the eye.

time after surgery. For a short time afterward, you'll need to wear an eye patch and apply medicated eyedrops to help the healing.

Full recovery may take weeks. When a vitrectomy is done for PDR with a massive vitreous hemorrhage, some blood may remain in the eye, or fresh bleeding may occur. It may take several weeks for your sight to clear.

Following a vitrectomy for traction retinal detachment or vitreous hemorrhage, vision improves in most people. When surgery fails to improve vision, it's usually because of irreparable damage to the retina from diabetes. But at times it can be due to complications of the surgery, recurring vitreous bleeding, retinal detachment or the formation of new blood vessels on the iris (neovascular glaucoma).

Self-care

There's no doubt that diabetic retinopathy is a serious disease. It's equally certain that you can take steps to slow its progression.

Control your blood sugar. Tight control of blood sugar slows the onset and progression of retinopathy and lessens the need for surgery. Tight control means keeping blood sugar levels as close to normal as possible. A normal range before eating is 70 to 110 milligrams of sugar per deciliter of blood (mg/dL), but that may not be realistic for many people. Another measure of good control is a result of 8 percent or less on a glycated hemoglobin test (hemoglobin A-1C test), which measures how well you've controlled your blood sugar level over the previous 2 to 3 months.

Tight control isn't possible for everyone, including some older adults, young children and people with cardiovascular disease. Talk to your doctor, endocrinologist or diabetes educator about the best management plan for you. A plan frequently involves:

- Taking insulin or other medications
- Monitoring blood sugar levels
- Following a healthy eating plan
- Getting regular exercise
- Maintaining a healthy weight

It may take some time before the benefits of lowering your blood sugar are realized. And it's important to note that better control lowers but doesn't eliminate your risk of developing retinopathy.

Keep an eye on vision changes. In addition to getting an annual eye exam, be alert to any sudden changes in your vision. Have your eyes checked promptly if you experience:

- Vision changes that last more than a few days or aren't associated with a change in blood sugar
- Eye pain, redness, floaters or light flashes

Keep your blood pressure down. Studies show that lowering blood pressure may slow the progression of diabetic retinopathy. To reduce your blood pressure, you may need to take medications or make lifestyle changes.

Stop smoking. Smoking is especially bad for people with diabetes because it promotes the closure of blood vessels.

Get support if you need it. Diabetes can take an emotional as well as physical toll. Stress, depression and anxiety are common among people with diabetes. In turn stress can cause swings in blood sugar levels. Don't hesitate to seek help from a counselor, therapist or support group. Relaxation techniques such as meditation also may be helpful.

Chapter 9

Retinal detachment

Retinal detachment is a serious eye condition that almost always leads to blindness if not treated promptly. Each year the condition affects about 30,000 people in the United States. The good news is that warning signs often appear before retinal detachment occurs. If these signs are heeded, early diagnosis of the condition and treatment by an ophthalmologist can save your vision.

What is retinal detachment? The retina is the light-sensitive tissue that lies smoothly against the inside back wall of your eye. Underneath the retina is the choroid, a thin layer of blood vessels that supplies oxygen and nutrients to the retina. Retinal detachment occurs when the retina separates from this underlying layer of blood vessels. Unless the detached retina is surgically reattached, you may permanently lose your vision in the affected eye .

Floaters, flashes and retinal detachments

At the root of this eye disorder are changes to the jellylike vitreous that fills the vitreous cavity of your eye. Over time your vitreous may change in consistency and partially liquefy. It may also begin to shrink. The partial liquefaction may progress to a point where the vitreous sags and separates from the surface of the retina. This is called posterior vitreous detachment (PVD), or vitreous collapse. It's a common condition and occurs to some extent in most people's eyes as they age.

PVD usually doesn't cause serious problems. The shifting or sagging vitreous may cause the appearance of new or different floaters in your field of vision. What looks like spots, specks, hairs and strings actually are small clumps of gel, fibers and cells floating in the vitreous. And what you're seeing are the shadows that this material casts on the retina. Common floaters appear gradually over time and, while annoying, are rarely a problem. They hardly ever require treatment.

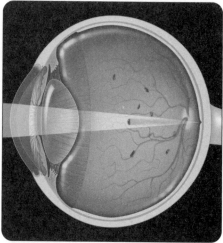

Floaters
Floaters can obstruct vision by intercepting light passing through the eye, casting a shadow on the retina.

If the vitreous pulls on the retina as it shifts and sags, you may see flashes of sparkling lights (photopsia) when your eyes are closed or you're in a darkened room. The phenomenon lasts for only a few seconds.

However, floaters and flashes can signal a more serious eye problem, particularly if they appear suddenly and with great intensity. When the pull of a sagging vitreous is strong enough, the retina may tear, leaving what looks like a small, jagged flap in the retina. Most tears occur along the periphery of the retina. That's

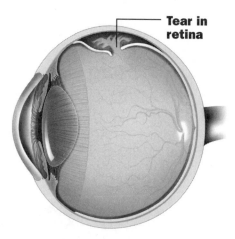

Tear in retina

Retinal detachment
When partially liquefied vitreous leaks through tears or holes, the retina may start to pull away from the underlying choroid layer. As more liquid accumulates, the detachment may expand, and parts of your visual field are blurred or lost.

where the vitreous is more firmly attached and can't separate without tugging hard. Such tears can lead to retinal detachment.

Retinal detachment occurs when vitreous liquid starts to leak under the retina at places opened by the tears. Leakage can also occur at tiny holes where the retina has thinned due to aging or other retinal disorders. As liquid collects, the areas of the retina surrounding these defects may begin to peel away from the underlying layer, the choroid (see figure 16 in the color section). Over time these detached areas may expand, like wallpaper that, once torn, slowly peels off a wall. The areas where the retina is detached lose their ability to see.

Not all tears and holes in the retina lead to retinal detachment. Sometimes the retina by these defects remains attached to the choroid relatively well. But detachment that goes undetected and untreated can progress and eventually involve the entire retina with complete loss of vision.

Signs and symptoms

Retinal detachment is painless, but visual symptoms almost always appear before it occurs. Here are some warning signs:

- The sudden appearance of many floaters
- A sensation of flashing lights that usually occurs in one eye but can be in both eyes at the same time
- A shadow over a portion of your visual field
- Blurred vision

Because most tears occur along the periphery of the retina, blurring may be noticeable initially in your peripheral vision.

When your retina tears, small blood vessels may be broken, letting blood seep into the vitreous and causing hazy vision or specks that appear to float before your eyes. If the floaters appear suddenly as a cloud of spots or a spider web and are accompanied by flashes of light, see your ophthalmologist immediately — you may have the beginnings of a retinal detachment. Prompt ophthalmologic attention is necessary to save your vision.

Risk factors

Your risk of developing a detached retina generally increases with age simply because the vitreous changes as you grow older. You're also at greater risk if you have had a previous retinal detachment in one eye or a family history of retinal detachment or are:

- Nearsighted (myopic)
- Male
- White

The following factors can cause the vitreous to pull at and tear the retina, so they also increase your risk of retinal detachment:

- Previous eye surgery (for example, cataract removal)
- Previous severe eye injury
- Weak areas in the periphery of your retina

Screening and diagnosis

An ophthalmologist can determine if you have a retinal hole, tear or detachment by looking carefully at the retina with an ophthalmoscope. If blood in your vitreous cavity prevents a clear view of the retina, he or she might also use sound waves (ultrasonography) to get a precise picture of your retina (see the sidebar "Vitreous hemorrhage and retinal detachment").

Treatment

Surgery is the only effective therapy for a retinal tear, hole or detachment. If a tear or a hole is treated before detachment develops, or if a retinal detachment is treated before the macula (the central part of the retina) detaches, you'll probably retain much of your vision.

Surgery for retinal tears

When a retinal tear or hole hasn't yet progressed to detachment, your eye surgeon may suggest one of two outpatient procedures: photocoagulation or cryopexy. Both methods can prevent the devel-

Vitreous hemorrhage and retinal detachment

A vitreous hemorrhage occurs when blood spills into the vitreous cavity from torn blood vessels in the retina. The torn vessels may accompany the formation of a retinal tear. Retinal detachment in the presence of a vitreous hemorrhage is hard to diagnose and treat because blood clouds the vitreous and prevents the surgeon from viewing the retina and locating the tear. When this happens the surgeon uses ultrasonography to diagnose the retinal detachment.

Ultrasonography is a painless test that sends sound waves through the hemorrhage to bounce off the retina. The returning sound waves create an image on a monitor that allows the doctor to determine the condition of the retina and other structures inside the eye. If a retinal detachment is found, you'll need a vitrectomy to remove the blood before the surgeon can repair the detachment.

In this situation you're at high risk of developing scar tissue in the vitreous and on the retina, a condition called proliferative vitreoretinopathy (PVR). PVR occurs when scar tissue folds or puckers the retina like wrinkled aluminum foil and prevents the retina from being reattached by pneumatic retinopexy or scleral buckling surgery alone.

opment of a retinal detachment in most cases. Healing typically takes from 10 to 14 days. Your vision may be blurred briefly following either procedure.

Photocoagulation. During photocoagulation (see pages 121 to 123) the surgeon directs a laser beam through a special contact lens to make burns around the retinal tear. The burns cause scarring, which usually holds the retina to the underlying tissue. This procedure requires no surgical incision, and it causes less irritation to the eye than does cryopexy.

Cryopexy. With cryopexy the surgeon uses intense cold to freeze the retina around the retinal tear. After a local anesthetic numbs your eye, a freezing probe is applied to the outer surface of the eye directly over the retinal defect. This freezing produces an inflammation that leads to the formation of a scar (much like with photo-coagulation), which seals the hole and holds the retina to the under-lying tissue. Cryopexy is used in instances where the tears are more difficult to reach with a laser, generally along the retinal periphery. Your eye may be red and swollen for some time after cryopexy.

Surgery for retinal detachment

Three different surgical procedures are commonly used to repair a retinal detachment: pneumatic retinopexy, scleral buckling and vitrectomy. Some of these procedures are done in conjunction with cryopexy. The purpose of these treatments is to close any retinal holes or tears and to reduce the tug on the retina from a shrinking vitreous. The severity and complexity of your condition will deter-mine which procedure your eye surgeon recommends.

Pneumatic retinopexy. Pneumatic retinopexy is a surgical tech-nique used for an uncomplicated detachment when the tear is located in the upper half of the retina. It's done on an outpatient basis using local anesthesia. First the surgeon performs cryopexy around the retinal tear. Then he or she withdraws a small amount of fluid from the anterior chamber to soften the eye and injects a bubble of expandable gas into the vitreous cavity. Over the next several days, the gas bubble expands, sealing the retinal tear by pushing against it and the detached area that surrounds the tear. With no new fluid passing through the retinal tear, fluid that had previously collected under the retina is absorbed, and the retina is able to reattach itself to the back wall of the eye.

Following surgery. You may have to hold your head in a cocked position for a few days after surgery, to make sure the gas bubble seals the retinal tear. It takes 2 to 6 weeks for the bubble to disap-pear. Until the gas is gone from your eye, you have to avoid lying or sleeping on your back. This keeps the bubble away from your lens and reduces the risk of cataract formation or a sudden pressure increase in your eye.

During that time you can't travel by airplane or be at a high alti-tude because a sudden drop in pressure would cause the gas bubble to expand rapidly, resulting in dangerously high pressure in your eye. Check with your surgeon on when this danger has passed.

The success rate of pneumatic retinopexy isn't as good as that of scleral buckling (described below). However, it can avoid a trip to the operating room and the need for incisional (cutting) surgery.

Complications. The complications of pneumatic retinopexy may include:
- Recurring retinal detachment
- Excessive scar tissue formation in the vitreous and retina
- Cataracts
- Glaucoma
- Gas getting under the retina
- Infection

These complications are rare, but if they do occur and go untreated, they can cause severe loss of vision. A recurring retinal detachment can usually be repaired with scleral buckling or vitrectomy.

Scleral buckling. Scleral buckling is the most common surgery for repairing retinal detachment. It's usually done in an operating room under local or general anesthesia. If you have an uncomplicated retinal detachment, this surgery may be done on an outpatient basis.

First the surgeon opens the conjunctiva and treats the retinal tears or holes with cryopexy. Then he or she indents (buckles) the sclera over the affected area by pressing in with a piece of silicone. The silicone material is either in the form of a soft sponge or a solid piece. The buckle closes the tear and helps reduce the circumference of the eyeball, thereby preventing further vitreous pulling and separation. When you have several tears or holes or an extensive detachment, the surgeon may create an encircling scleral buckle around the entire circumference of the eye.

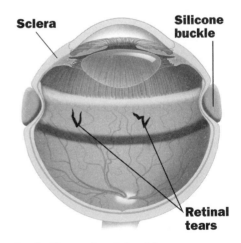

Sclera

Silicone buckle

Retinal tears

Encircling scleral buckle
Silicone indents or buckles the sclera, thereby reducing the size of the eyeball and the amount of traction put on the retina by a shrinking vitreous. The silicone piece is stitched permanently to the outside of the eye.

The scleral buckle is stitched to the outer surface of the sclera. Before tying the sutures holding the buckle in place, the surgeon may make a small cut in the sclera and drain any fluid that has collected under the detached retina. The buckle is then covered with the conjunctiva. Once the incision heals, there is little evidence of the operation, and the buckle remains in place for the rest of your life. Some surgeons may choose a temporary buckle for simple retinal detachments, using a small rubber balloon that's inflated and later removed.

Repairing retinal detachment with scleral buckling works more than 80 percent of the time with one operation. But a reattached retina doesn't guarantee normal vision. How well you see following surgery depends in part on whether the macula was affected by the detachment before surgery, and if it was, for how long. Your sight isn't likely to return to normal if the macula was detached. Even if the macula wasn't affected and scleral buckling successfully repairs your retina, you have a 10 percent chance of losing some vision due to wrinkling, or puckering, of the macula.

If the first operation fails, your doctor usually can try to reattach the retina with one or more additional operations. Additional surgery increases the rate of successful reattachment to more than 90 percent.

Scarring. Scleral buckling is generally successful, but sometimes — in approximately 5 percent to 10 percent of the procedures — the retina fails to reattach to the choroid. This is often due to the formation of scar tissue on the retinal surface. Scar tissue present even before the operation can pull on the retina and prevent it from reattaching. The pull of scar tissue that forms after the operation can cause the retina to separate again after having been attached during surgery. This usually happens 1 to 2 months following surgery.

This condition is treated by removing the scar tissue with a procedure called a vitrectomy (see page 135) and redoing the scleral buckling. In some complicated cases, the surgeon injects air, other gases or silicone oil into the vitreous cavity to push the retina back against the wall of the eye. Eventually your eye absorbs the air or gas and replaces it with fluid that the eye normally produces. Silicone, however, doesn't get absorbed and has to be removed once the retina is reattached and healed completely.

Complications. Complications occur infrequently but should be mentioned. Any one of them can result in the need for more surgery, the loss of some or all vision in the eye that was operated on, or in rare instances, the loss of that eye. They are:

- Bleeding under the retina or into the vitreous cavity. This can occur while subretinal fluid is being drained or when a buckle suture inadvertently perforates the sclera and enters the eye.
- Increased pressure inside your eyeball (glaucoma). This is due to a swelling of the choroid and narrowing of the angle in the anterior chamber.
- Double vision (diplopia). This is caused by interference from the buckle with the function of muscles that keep your eyes aligned. It may be temporary. If it's not it may require corrective glasses or surgery on the eye muscles.

Vitrectomy. Occasionally, bleeding or inflammation clouds the vitreous and blocks the surgeon's view of the detached retina. In other instances scar tissue makes it impossible to repair a retinal detachment with pneumatic retinopexy or scleral buckling alone. In these situations a procedure called vitrectomy (see pages 123 to 125) can remove the clouded vitreous or scar tissue.

The surgeon accomplishes this with a variety of delicate instruments passed into the eyeball through small openings in the sclera. These instruments include a light probe that illuminates the inside of the eye, a cutter to remove vitreous or scar tissue and an infusion tube that replaces the volume of removed tissue with a balanced salt solution to maintain the normal pressure and shape of the eye.

After the vitrectomy is completed, the surgeon performs the scleral buckling procedure and may fill the inside of your eye with air, gas or silicone oil to help seal the retina against the wall of the eye.

Vitrectomy may also be performed for conditions other than complicated retinal detachments, including:

- Vitreous clouding by blood that prevents light from reaching the retina
- Macular puckers (epiretinal membranes)
- Infection inside the eye (endophthalmitis)
- A foreign body inside the eye

Vitrectomy surgery typically lasts 1 to 2 hours but may take significantly longer in more complex cases. The complex cases are often done under general anesthesia, and shorter procedures are usually performed under local anesthesia.

Following surgery. You can experience some discomfort and a scratchy sensation in your eye. Severe pain is unlikely. If it does occur, let your surgeon know immediately. You can expect your eye to be red, swollen, watery and slightly sore for up to a month following any of the surgical procedures described above. Wearing an eye patch may provide some relief. Your doctor may also prescribe antibacterial or dilating eyedrops to help the healing process. You'll have to avoid strenuous activities during this time. It'll take about 8 to 10 weeks for your eye to heal fully. Then your doctor will examine your eyes to determine your postoperative vision and, if you wear eyeglasses, whether you need a new prescription.

Your vision may take many months to improve following surgery to repair a complicated retinal detachment. Some people don't recover any lost vision.

Complications. The complications of vitrectomy are similar to those for other types of retinal detachment surgery. They include a retinal tear, redetachment of the retina, a cataract or an infection. Any of these complications can lead to partial or complete loss of vision in the affected eye or, rarely, loss of the eye itself. How much vision you retain will depend on the severity of the detachment.

Prompt action can save your sight

If you notice the warning signs of a retinal detachment, talk with your ophthalmologist immediately. Prompt action can save your vision. Your ophthalmologist can tell you about the various risks and benefits of all your treatment options. Together you can determine what treatment is appropriate for you.

Chapter 10

Age-related macular degeneration

Age-related macular degeneration (AMD) is a chronic disease that occurs when tissue in the macula, the part of your retina that's responsible for central vision, deteriorates. The result is blurred central vision or a blind spot in the center of your visual field. This condition tends to develop as you get older, hence the "age-related" part of its name. Macular degeneration is the leading cause of severe vision loss in people age 50 and older.

The first sign of AMD may be a need for more light when you do close-up work. Fine newsprint may become harder to read and street signs more difficult to recognize. Eventually you may notice that when you're looking at an object, what should be a smooth, straight line appears distorted or crooked. Gray or blank spots may mask the center of your visual field. The condition may progress rapidly, leading to severe vision loss in one or both eyes.

Macular degeneration affects your central vision but not peripheral vision; thus it does not cause total blindness. Still, the loss of clear central vision — critical for reading, driving, recognizing people's faces and doing detail work — greatly affects your quality of life. In most cases the damage caused by macular degeneration can't be reversed, but early detection may help reduce the extent of vision loss.

Types

There are two types of macular degeneration: dry macular degeneration and wet macular degeneration. To understand the differences between these two forms of the disease, it's also important to understand what they have in common. The macula is the center of your retina and is made up of densely packed light-sensitive cells called cones and rods. These cells, particularly the cones, are essential for central vision. The choroid is an underlying layer of blood vessels that nourishes the cones and rods of the retina. A layer of tissue forming the outermost surface of the retina is called the retinal pigment epithelium (RPE). The RPE is a critical passageway for nutrients from the choroid to the retina and helps remove waste products from the retina to the choroid.

As you age, the RPE may deteriorate and thin (a process known as atrophy), which sets off a chain of events. The nutritional and waste-removing cycles between the retina and the choroid are interrupted. Waste deposits begin to form. Lacking nutrients, the light-sensitive cells of the macula become damaged. The damaged cells can no longer send normal signals through the optic nerve to your brain, and your vision becomes blurred. This is often the first symptom of macular degeneration.

Dry macular degeneration

Most people with macular degeneration have the dry form. In fact, AMD always starts out as the dry form. Dry AMD may initially affect only one eye but, in most cases, both eyes eventually become involved.

Dry macular degeneration occurs when the RPE cells begin to thin. The normally uniform reddish color of the macula takes on a mottled appearance. Drusen, which look like yellow dots, appear under the retina (see figure 13 in the color section).

Initially, in spite of these developments, you may notice little or no change in your vision. Many people who've received a diagnosis of early-stage dry macular degeneration may not be bothered with symptoms such as blurred eyesight until they live to a very old age. But as the drusen and mottled pigmentation continue to develop, your vision may deteriorate sooner. Thinning of the RPE may progress to a point where this protective layer of the retina disappears (see figure 14 in the color section). This affects the overlying cones and rods and may result in complete loss of your central vision.

Wet macular degeneration

The wet form of macular degeneration accounts for 10 percent to 15 percent of all cases, but it's responsible for nearly 90 percent of the severe vision loss that people with AMD experience. If you develop wet macular degeneration in one eye, your odds of getting it in the other eye increase greatly.

Wet macular degeneration develops when new blood vessels grow from the choroid underneath the macula. These vessels leak fluid or blood — hence it is called wet AMD — and cause your central vision to blur. All eyes with wet AMD also show signs of dry AMD, that is, drusen and mottled pigmentation of the retina (see figure 15 in the color section). In addition, what should be straight lines in your sight become wavy or crooked, and blank spots appear in your field of vision. Sight loss is usually rapid and severe, resulting in

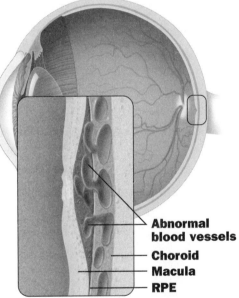

Abnormal blood vessels

Choroid

Macula

RPE

Wet macular degeneration
Abnormal blood vessels growing out of the choroid push up the retinal pigment epithelium (RPE). Fluid and blood leaking from these vessels can cause severe sight loss.

legal blindness, defined as 20/200 vision or worse. This means that what someone with normal vision can see from 200 feet, a person with 20/200 vision can see only from 20 feet.

A comparatively rare form of wet macular degeneration is called retinal pigment epithelial detachment (PED). In this instance fluid leaks from the choroid although no abnormal blood vessels have started to grow there. The fluid collects under the retinal pigment epithelium, causing what looks like a blister or a bump under the macula. This kind of macular degeneration causes the same symptoms as wet AMD and frequently progresses to wet AMD with newly growing abnormal blood vessels.

Signs and symptoms

Macular degeneration usually develops gradually and painlessly. The signs and symptoms of the disease may vary, depending on the type of macular degeneration you have.

With dry macular degeneration you may notice the following symptoms:

- The need for increasingly bright illumination when reading or doing close work
- Printed words that appear increasingly blurry
- Colors that seem washed out and dull
- A gradual increase in the haziness of your overall vision
- A blind spot in the center of your visual field combined with a profound drop in your central vision

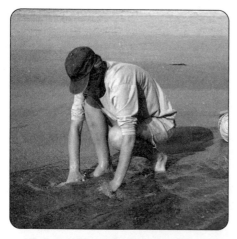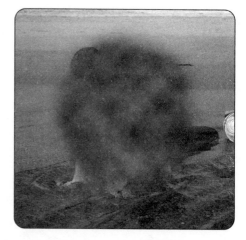

Vision with macular degeneration
As macular degeneration develops, your eyesight becomes impaired by general haziness and a blind spot at the center of your visual field.

With wet macular degeneration, the following symptoms may appear rapidly:

- Visual distortions, such as straight lines appearing wavy or crooked (a doorway or street sign that seems out of whack)
- Decreased central vision
- A central blurry spot

In either form of macular degeneration, your vision may falter in one eye while the other remains fine for years. You may not notice any or much change because your good eye compensates for the weak one. It's when the condition develops in both eyes that your vision and lifestyle are dramatically affected.

Causes

Generally speaking, macular degeneration involves a breakdown in the system that provides nourishment to and removes waste from the macula. Although this breakdown often accompanies a deterioration of the RPE, the reasons why the system stops working are poorly understood. The disease is likely triggered by a combination of several factors.

Dry macular degeneration

Dry macular degeneration is the result of a deterioration of the retinal pigment epithelium brought on by aging. The light-sensitive cells of the macula continuously shed used-up outer segments as waste. This waste is broken down and disposed of by the RPE into the choroid. At the same time, cones and rods continuously produce new outer segments to replace the discarded ones.

When you develop dry macular degeneration, the waste disposal system falls apart. Aging slows the process to a point where waste starts to accumulate in the RPE. This accumulation interferes with the normal function of the RPE, causing the light-sensitive cells of the macula to degenerate.

The appearance of mottled pigmentation and drusen — which are clumps of waste deposit — signals this development. The appearance of small drusen can be common as you age and does not interfere with vision, but large drusen with indistinct edges are often associated with a decrease in vision.

Wet macular degeneration

In wet macular degeneration, abnormal blood vessels grow from the choroid underneath the retinal pigment epithelium. This is called choroidal neovascularization (CNV). Think of tree roots growing under a sidewalk and lifting it up. These abnormal blood vessels may leak fluid and blood, lifting up the RPE and the macula in blisters or bumps. This damages the light-sensitive cells of the macula. Eventually the abnormal blood vessels transform into scar tissue, creating a permanent blind spot in the center of your vision.

Much like the dry form of macular degeneration, a breakdown in the waste removal system may be what's causing the CNV. When the waste from the cones and rods is not disposed of and begins to accumulate, sufficient flow of nutrients to the macula is interrupted. The abnormal growth of blood vessels may be a response to this interruption in the flow of nutrients. And without enough nutrients, healthy tissue in the macula begins to deteriorate.

Risk factors

Researchers may not know the exact causes of macular degeneration, but they have identified some contributing factors. They include:

- Age
- Race
- Sex
- Light-colored eyes
- A family history of macular degeneration
- Long-term exposure to ultraviolet light and blue light (the wavelength just above ultraviolet), which includes sunlamps as well as regular sunlight
- Low blood levels of minerals and antioxidant vitamins, such as A, C and E
- Cigarette smoking

- Cardiovascular disease — for example, circulatory problems, stroke, heart attack, angina

Age and race figure prominently in the development of macular degeneration. In the United States the disease is most common in whites over age 50. It affects about 11 percent of whites ages 65 to 74, and 28 percent of whites age 75 and older. Macular degeneration is less common in blacks, Asian-Americans and American Indians than it is in other groups.

Having a family history of macular degeneration is perhaps the greatest risk factor. Women are more likely than are men to develop macular degeneration and, because they tend to live longer, to suffer the effects of severe vision loss from the disease.

Exposure to environmental pollution — especially cigarette smoke — greatly increases your risk. Smokers are two to three times more likely to develop macular degeneration than are non-smokers.

Screening and diagnosis

Age-related macular degeneration (AMD) is diagnosed with a thorough eye examination. If you notice any changes in your central vision or your ability to see colors and fine detail, particularly if

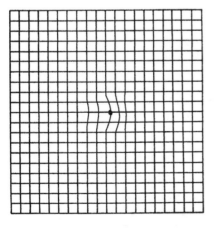 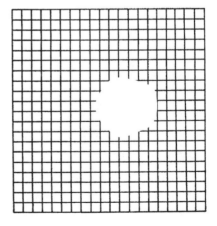

Indications of AMD on an Amsler grid
Someone in the early stages of macular degeneration may see distorted grid lines (left).
Someone at a more advanced stage may see a blank spot at the center of the grid (right).

you're over age 50, it's advisable to see your eye doctor. One of the things he or she looks for while examining the inside of your eye is the presence of drusen and mottled pigmentation in the macula.

The eye examination includes a simple test of your central vision using an Amsler grid (see page 143). If you have macular degeneration, when you look at the grid some of the straight lines may seem faded, broken or distorted. By noting where the break or distortion occurs — usually on or near the center of the grid — your eye doctor can better determine the location and extent of your macular damage.

This helpful test can be done outside a doctor's office. If you're looking for early symptoms of macular degeneration, you can administer the test yourself at home (see "Screening your vision" on page 148).

To evaluate the extent of the damage from macular degeneration, your eye doctor may use fluorescein angiography. In this procedure he or she injects fluorescent dye into a vein in your arm and takes photographs as the dye passes through blood vessels in your retina and choroid. Your doctor then uses these photographs to detect changes in macular pigmentation or the existence of abnormal blood vessels in your macula that may not be visible to the bare eye.

Treatment

Currently there's no treatment for dry macular degeneration. However, this doesn't mean you'll eventually lose all of your sight. Dry macular degeneration usually progresses slowly, so many people with this condition are able to live relatively normal, productive lives, especially if only one eye is affected.

If you have wet macular degeneration, some treatment options are available. But the success of the treatment depends on the location and the extent of the abnormal blood vessels, or choroidal neovascularization (CNV). Be aware that successful treatment means stopping further progress of the disease. In most cases the damage already caused by AMD can't be reversed. The sooner CNV is detected, the better your chances of treatment preserving what's left of your central vision.

The three treatments currently available are photocoagulation, photodynamic therapy (PDT) and macular translocation surgery, each of which can be done as an outpatient procedure. Experimental procedures using an infrared laser (transpupillary thermotherapy, or TTT) or radiation therapy are being tested but are still unproven to benefit people with macular degeneration.

Photocoagulation

Photocoagulation can seal off and destroy the CNV that has developed under your macula. (For a detailed description of this procedure, see pages 121 to 123.) It can prevent further damage to the macula and halt continued vision loss. Only about 20 percent of people who have wet macular degeneration are candidates for this procedure. Whether it's right for you depends on the location and appearance of the CNV, the amount of blood that has leaked, and the general health of your macula. Even if photocoagulation is a viable option for you, the results can be disappointing. Laser surgery to destroy the CNV is successful only about 50 percent of the time. And even successfully destroyed CNV has a tendency to recur. Repeat laser treatment may not be possible in such an event.

If you noticed a dark or gray spot in or near your central vision before laser treatment, the procedure will make vision in that spot completely and permanently blank. With time you may not notice the blank spot any longer, especially when you use both eyes. And if you closely monitor your vision and have frequent follow-ups with your doctor, you're likely to retain more sight than if you had received no treatment at all. Photocoagulation is the only proven treatment for CNV when it's not located directly under the fovea at the center of your macula.

Photodynamic therapy

Photodynamic therapy (PDT) is a new treatment for CNV that's located directly under the fovea. The fovea lies at the center of your macula and in healthy eyes provides your sharpest vision. If conventional hot-laser surgery were used at this location, it would destroy all central vision. PDT increases your chances of preserving some of that vision.

This procedure combines a cold laser and a light-sensitizing drug that's injected into your bloodstream. The drug concentrates in the CNV under the macula. When the doctor directs cold laser light at it, the drug releases substances that close off the abnormal blood vessels without damaging the macula, and the CNV transforms into a thin scar. The overlying rods and cones are largely preserved, resulting in better vision than if you had had hot-laser surgery or no treatment at all. The therapy can be repeated if the CNV doesn't close or if it reopens after initial closure.

The Food and Drug Administration recently approved the drug verteporfin (Visudyne) for use in photodynamic therapy. Studies involving verteporfin demonstrate that over a 2-year period, multiple treatment sessions reduced vision loss for two-thirds of the people who had clearly defined CNV under the fovea. Though these results are promising, other long-term benefits are still under study. For example, further research will determine if this treatment also helps people who have poorly defined or hidden areas of CNV.

Macular translocation surgery

Macular translocation surgery is an experimental treatment for wet macular degeneration. This surgery can be used if the abnormal blood vessels are located directly under the fovea. To start the procedure, the surgeon detaches the retina, shifts the fovea away from the CNV and relocates it over healthy tissue. When the CNV is exposed, the surgeon can then use a hot laser to destroy blood vessels without damaging the fovea. This surgery can be performed only if your vision loss is recent (usually within 1 to 3 months), the extent of CNV is limited and the tissue around the fovea is healthy.

Prevention

Nothing you do can change your race or genetic makeup or keep you from getting older — all major risk factors for macular degeneration. But preliminary evidence suggests that any of the following measures may help prevent or delay the development of macular degeneration. These measures are best started before macular degeneration develops and your vision starts to decrease:

- Research indicates that people at high risk of the advanced stages of macular degeneration were able to lower that risk with a dietary supplement of antioxidants, zinc and copper (see pages 62 to 63). Antioxidants are substances that prevent oxidative damage to tissue such as the retina. Foods with antioxidants are those rich in vitamins A, C and E. And it helps to eat a nutritionally balanced, low-fat diet containing five or more servings of fruits and vegetables every day.
- The antioxidants lutein and zeaxanthin are nutrients found in high concentrations in egg yolk, corn and spinach. Preliminary studies show that high levels of lutein and zeaxanthin in your blood may protect your retina.
- Wear sunglasses that block out harmful ultraviolet light. Orange-, yellow- or amber-tinted lenses can filter out both ultraviolet light and blue light that may damage your retina.
- Stop smoking. Smokers are two to three times more likely to develop macular degeneration than are nonsmokers. Ask your doctor for help to stop smoking.
- Manage your other diseases. For example, if you have cardiovascular disease, take your medication and follow your doctor's instructions for controlling the condition. If it's not well controlled, it may contribute to the onset of macular degeneration.
- Get regular eye exams. Early detection of macular degeneration increases your chances of preventing serious vision loss. If you're over the age of 50, get an exam every 2 to 5 years. If you have a family history of macular degeneration, have your eyes examined more frequently, perhaps annually.
- Screen your vision regularly. If you've received a diagnosis of early-stage macular degeneration, your doctor may suggest that you regularly monitor your vision at home with an Amsler grid (see "Screening your vision" on page 148). Doing so may enable you to detect subtle changes in your vision at the earliest possible time and seek help promptly.

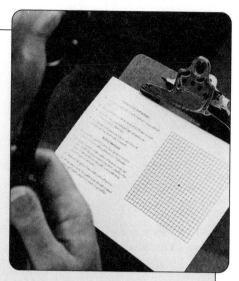

Screening your vision

You can check your vision using an Amsler grid. This simple test may help you detect changes in your sight that you otherwise may not notice. You can perform the test with the grid in hand, as shown at right, or hang the grid someplace where you'll see it often — on your refrigerator or bathroom mirror, for instance.

Here's what you do:

- Hold the grid 14 inches in front of you in good light. You need to use your reading glasses if you normally wear them.
- Cover one eye.
- Look directly at the center dot with the uncovered eye.
- While looking at this dot, see whether all of the lines of the grid are straight, complete and of the same contrast.
- Repeat steps 1 through 4 with the other eye.
- If any part of the grid is missing or looks wavy, blurred or dark, contact your ophthalmologist immediately.

If you have some vision loss owing to macular degeneration, your eye doctor can prescribe optical devices called low-vision aids that will help you see better for close-up work. Or your doctor may refer you to a low-vision specialist. In addition a wide variety of support services and rehabilitation programs are available that may help you adjust your lifestyle. The next chapter more fully outlines ways of coping with low vision.

Chapter 11

Living with low vision

Several of the preceding chapters in this book explain how various eye diseases are diagnosed and treated. Although prompt treatment can stop or minimize further damage to your eyes, it doesn't always recover vision that was damaged in the early stages of the disease, before the disease was diagnosed. In some cases this damage can be extensive. With glaucoma, for example, your peripheral vision can be almost completely lost before you realize something is wrong.

This vision loss may prevent you from doing many everyday tasks or participating in activities you enjoy. You may not be able to read print, see the numbers on your telephone clearly, perform necessary tasks at your job or move around the house safely. Your eyes may not be able to adjust to contrast or glare. You may not be able to distinguish colors. Your vision loss may be owing to a single problem or several problems in combination. The effects can range from mild to severe.

When this happens you may have what is known as low vision. Having low vision means your eye condition can't be corrected with standard eyeglasses, contact lenses or surgery. Low vision is often the result of conditions such as macular degeneration, glaucoma or diabetic retinopathy. It can also be the result of serious eye injuries or birth defects.

Warning signs that you may have low vision

Remember that low vision is determined by the degree to which vision problems interfere with your everyday needs and activities. Some of these problems are listed below:

- Difficulty recognizing the faces of relatives and friends
- Problems doing close-up work, including reading, cooking and sewing
- Problems picking out and matching the color of your clothes
- Difficulty seeing because lights seem dimmer than they used to
- Trouble reading street, bus or store signs

It is important that you consult an eye doctor or low-vision specialist about your vision problems. He or she can help assess what you need to do in order to function independently. Your eye doctor can also recommend various vision services and resources that may be of use to you.

Source: National Eye Institute Web site, 2000

Low-vision rehabilitation

Sometimes people with low vision believe that nothing else can be done to improve the way they perform daily living skills. The reality is that many types of vision loss respond well to low-vision rehabilitation, which may help you resume an active, independent life within the limitations of your particular eye condition.

Rehabilitation starts with an assessment by a low-vision specialist. The low-vision specialist is an eye doctor trained in evaluating people with low vision. This eye specialist may also work with other health care professionals, such as social workers, occupational therapists and others to maximize your remaining vision.

Low-vision rehabilitation uses low-vision aids, proper lighting, and special training to help you resume normal activities. When you see a low-vision specialist, he or she compiles a complete history of your vision problem and may ask you to describe the tasks you're having difficulty performing. He or she then decides on a course of testing. During this testing, low-vision aids including glasses, magnifiers, telescopes and electronic devices, as well as nonoptical devices such as reading stands and lamps, are tried out and reviewed.

This testing is not just a trial-and-error process, although sometimes it may seem that way. Sometimes testing must be done over several visits — as this process takes time — and can be fatiguing. But the low-vision examination is carried out in a manner designed to maximize your vision and achieve the goals set by you and your doctor at the start of testing.

Once the low-vision specialist determines the best aids for you, he or she develops a training program. The program may be carried out by the specialist with his or her staff or by another professional, such as a vision rehabilitation specialist, who can teach you how to use low-vision aids and provide special training. This training is important because as simple as these aids may seem, if they're not used properly, they won't function in the way they're intended to. Just as someone who has had physical trauma or a stroke may need rehabilitation to learn to do simple tasks again, people with low vision also may need to learn to do things in a slightly different way.

Low-vision aids

An array of low-vision aids is available, including everything from magnifying devices and enlarged telephone dials to closed-circuit television and machines that talk. A low-vision specialist will help you find the device, or perhaps several devices, tailored to your specific vision problem. These devices are generally affordable and easy to use.

Optical devices

These low-vision aids can help you use your remaining vision more effectively. They're frequently used in conjunction with regular prescription glasses. They include magnifiers for close-up work and telescopes for distance vision.

Magnifying eyeglasses. In magnifying eyeglasses a magnifying lens stronger than your regular prescription glasses is mounted in your eyeglass frames along with your regular lens, or it's mounted on a special headband. These glasses allow you to use both hands for close-up tasks, such as reading. You need to hold the reading material close to your eyes, which may be tiring. It may also be difficult to illuminate the page sufficiently. Plenty of light and a reading stand can help make you more comfortable and be easier on your posture.

Hand-held and stand magnifiers. Hand-held and stand magnifiers allow you to read print or work with objects positioned at a normal distance from your eyes. A hand-held magnifier is useful for reading price tags, labels and restaurant menus. The device is less practical for activities such as continuous reading because you have to hold the lens at a steady distance from the reading material, which can be exhausting. Stand magnifiers can be adjusted at a fixed distance directly above the object you're looking at. Hand-held and stand magnifiers are available with built-in light sources.

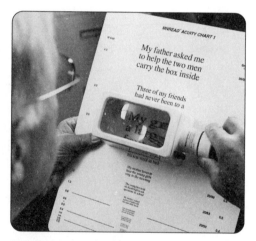

Hand-held magnifier

A low-vision specialist can help you choose the right type of magnifier with the correct strength or power for your particular vision problem. And remember, a magnifier is most effective when it's held at the correct distance. This requires testing at different positions to find the one that best serves your specific need.

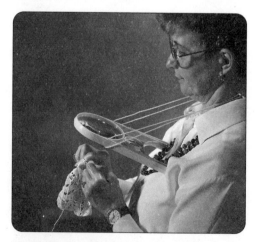

Neckstrap-supported magnifier

Thank you for purchasing *Mayo Clinic on Vision and Eye Health*

Thank you for purchasing *Mayo Clinic on Vision and Eye Health*. Please take a few minutes to complete this questionnaire. Your input will help us develop other books and products. We also can inform you of products that might be of interest to you.

As our way of saying thanks, we will send you a free issue of one of our highly acclaimed newsletters: *Mayo Clinic Health Letter* or *Mayo Clinic Women's HealthSource*. Please select **one** of the newsletters below:

☐ *Mayo Clinic Health Letter* is a monthly 8-page newsletter that covers general health issues and provides information you can use to live a healthier life.

☐ *Mayo Clinic Women's HealthSource* is a monthly 8-page newsletter that is devoted entirely to the special health interests of women.

1. Which of these health topics are you interested in? (*Please select up to 5 topics.*)

☐ Allergies or asthma
☐ Alzheimer's/memory disorders
☐ Arthritis
☐ Breast cancer
☐ Chronic pain
☐ Colon cancer
☐ Depression
☐ Diabetes
☐ Digestive diseases
☐ Eye or vision problems
☐ Hearing loss
☐ Heart disease
☐ High blood pressure
☐ Impotence or erectile dysfunction
☐ Lung cancer
☐ Menopause
☐ Migraines or other headaches
☐ Osteoporosis
☐ Pregnancy
☐ Prostate problems
☐ Stroke

2. Which of the following lifestyle topics are you interested in?

☐ Alternative medicine
☐ Exercise and fitness
☐ Healthy cooking
☐ Healthy aging
☐ Healthy weight
☐ Nutrition
☐ Skin care
☐ Stress management
☐ Vitamins, minerals or herbs

3. Where did you purchase this book?

☐ Book club
☐ Bookstore
☐ Discount store (e.g., *Kmart, Target*)
☐ Drugstore
☐ Gift
☐ Internet
☐ Mail order
☐ Phone order
☐ Retail store
☐ Warehouse store (*Sam's Club, etc.*)

4. What sources do you use to get health information?

☐ Books
☐ Internet
☐ Magazines
☐ Newsletters
☐ Television
☐ Other

5. Do you have access to the Internet?
☐ Yes   ☐ No

Name _____

Address _____ Apt _____

City _____ State _____ Zip _____

E-mail Address _____

Tell us where to send your FREE newsletter issue:

SRVY-12

BUSINESS REPLY MAIL

FIRST-CLASS MAIL   PERMIT NO. 251   ROCHESTER MN

POSTAGE WILL BE PAID BY ADDRESSEE

MAYO CLINIC HEALTH INFORMATION

CENTERPLACE 5

200 1ST ST SW

ROCHESTER MN   55902-9826

Telescopes. Conventional magnifying lenses don't help people with low vision see objects better at a distance, even objects that are just across the room. A telescope magnifies objects in the distance, but at the expense of a greatly narrowed field of vision. Telescopes may be held in the hand or mounted on eyeglasses. Hand-held telescopes are best used for short-term viewing, such as reading bus numbers or street signs. An eyeglass-mounted system is better for long-term viewing, for example, when you're watching television or an outdoor sporting event, or for when you need to use your hands for a close-up task.

Adaptive technology

Devices such as televisions or computers can be adapted to suit the special needs of people who otherwise may not be able to use them.

Closed-circuit televisions. Closed-circuit televisions, also known as CCTVs, help many people with low vision read books and newspapers, manage their checkbooks, read prescription bottles or look at photos. They provide much greater magnification than standard optical devices. There are many options to choose from.

A CCTV basically consists of a camera and a 12- or 19-inch monitor. You pass the material you want to read under the camera, which magnifies the print and displays it on the monitor. You can

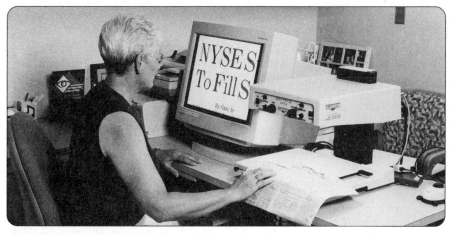

Closed-circuit television
Placing material such as a newspaper under the camera (right) allows you to read greatly magnified print on the monitor (left).

adjust the magnification to a type size that you can read comfortably. You can also adjust the color, brightness, contrast and background lighting of the screen to suit your needs.

Certain CCTVs can be connected to your computer. You only need one monitor because the computer and the CCTV can share the screen — one part of it shows computer files, the other displays CCTV material. Another type of CCTV allows you to scan large amounts of text that can be stored in the device and read on the monitor at a later time.

Portable CCTVs have a hand-held camera that you pass over materials to enlarge what you wish to see. You can view the enlarged material on a standard CCTV monitor, a small portable monitor or on the screen of your television set or computer monitor, depending on which option you choose.

Personal reading machines. A personal reading machine is formally referred to as an optical character recognition (OCR) system. It's a type of read-aloud device. The OCR operates something like a small photocopier — an internal camera scans print and then reads it aloud with a synthetic voice. OCRs can read almost anything that's printed, but they don't work with handwritten material.

You can use an OCR by itself or connect it to your computer. When it's linked to a computer, the scanned material can be converted into various forms, such as Braille, large print, voice or computer files.

Computer equipment and programs. Computer equipment and programs that enlarge text and images displayed on a computer monitor are available. These enable you to word process, use spreadsheets or browse the Internet — whatever you need to do on a computer at home or work.

A new, sophisticated and relatively expensive option involves installing a synthetic voice device on your computer. You can either use a synthesizer device or install a synthesizer program that uses your computer's existing sound system if it has one. Whichever synthesizer you have reads the text on your monitor using a computer-generated voice. It also tells you what's occurring on the screen: where the cursor is, what text is highlighted and other essential computer activities.

Other low-vision aids

Technology isn't the only tool
you can use to help you see better. Other available materials
and devices are simple and
easy to use. They include:

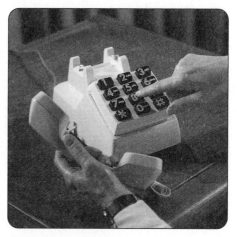

Enlarged telephone dial

- Large-print books, news-
  papers and magazines
- Check-writing guides
- Large playing cards
- Enlarged telephone dials
- Watches with high-con-
  trast faces
- Machines that talk, for
  example, timers and clocks

And don't forget one of the most important aids of all — adequate lighting. Even if you don't have a vision-limiting eye disorder, as you age you need more light to comfortably see than you
did when you were younger. Here are some lighting tips:

- When you're reading or doing other close-up work, choose a
  suitable lamp. One of the best is a desk or swing lamp that has
  an adjustable arm and provides 60 to 70 watts of incandescent
  light.
- Place your lamp about 4 to 8 inches from your reading material but off to the side a bit to reduce glare.
- Wear a visor or a hat with a wide brims to block annoying
  overhead light.
- Wear polarizing or tinted lenses to control glare.
- Use a piece of dark construction paper as a place holder and to
  reduce glare when you read.

Adaptive techniques

In addition to low-vision aids and proper lighting, other measures
can help you continue to lead an active life in spite of impaired
vision. Some ideas for daily living include:

- Use public transportation or ask family members for help with driving.
- Contact your local senior citizens agency for a list of vans and shuttles, volunteer driving networks or ride-shares.
- Optimize the vision you do have by using the best possible prescription for your glasses and keeping an extra pair handy.
- Tell friends and family members about your vision problems so that they can assist you with certain tasks.
- Don't become socially isolated. A common frustration is the inability to recognize people and greet them by name. If this happens to you, try asking acquaintances to say hello and state their name when they approach you so that you can greet them in return.
- Your eye doctor or low-vision specialist can refer you to government or private agencies for help. For more information see the appendix "Additional Resources."

Ask your doctor about receiving professional help to make your home more convenient for you to live in. Here are some tips for making your home and yard safer:

- Eliminate throw rugs and other tripping hazards.
- Install an intercom at your front door so that visitors can identify themselves.
- Install wireless sensor lights throughout the house so that you'll always have illumination, even if you leave during the day and come back at night. A less expensive option is to put an automatic night light in your entry area.
- Line all walkways in your yard with plants that differ sharply in color from the color of the walkway.
- Place low-voltage lighting along paths in your yard.
- Mark edges of stairs with paint or tape in a contrasting color.

Growing older does not necessarily mean poorer eyesight. Many older adults continue to maintain good vision. Nevertheless, it's a fact that people over the age of 65 are at greater risk of developing low vision. That makes vigilance — and regular eye examinations — even more important. It's also helpful to develop a partnership with your eye doctor or low-vision specialist to make the most of your vision.

Additional resources

Various organizations in your community may provide you with assistance and information about vision and eye health. Besides organizations directed specifically toward the blind and visually impaired, service organizations for older adults and people with disabilities also can help.

Some major national organizations associated with eye care are listed below, but these are not all of the resources available. The services these organizations may provide include instruction in independent home living, mobility training, counseling on living and coping with visual impairment, advice on locating eye specialists, transportation, talking books and other reading materials, and even recreational opportunities.

American Academy of Ophthalmology

P. O. Box 7424
San Francisco, CA 94120-7424
415-561-8500
www.aao.org

American Association of People With Disabilities

1819 H St. N.W., Suite 330
Washington, DC 20006
202-457-0046 or 800-840-8844
www.aapd.com

American Association of the Deaf-Blind

814 Thayer Ave., Suite 302
Silver Spring, MD 20910-4500
800-735-2258
www.tr.wosc.osshe.edu/dblink/aadb.htm

American Council of the Blind

1155 15th St. N.W., Suite 1004
Washington, DC 20005
202-467-5081 or 800-424-8666
www.acb.org

American Foundation for the Blind

11 Penn Plaza, Suite 300
New York, NY 10001-2018
212-502-7600 or 800-232-5463
www.afb.org

American Health Assistance Foundation

15825 Shady Grove Road, Suite 140
Rockville, MD 20850
301-948-3244 or 800-437-2423
www.ahaf.org

American Optometric Association

243 N. Lindbergh Blvd.
St. Louis, MO 63141
314-991-4100
www.aoanet.org

Association for Education and Rehabilitation of the Blind and Visually Impaired

4600 Duke St., Suite 430
P.O. Box 22397
Alexandria, VA 22304
703-823-9690
www.aerbvi.org

Association for Macular Diseases

210 E. 64th St., 8th Floor
New York, NY 10021
212-605-3719
www.macula.org

Foundation Fighting Blindness

11435 Cronhill Drive
Owings Mills, MD 21117-2220
410-568-0150 or 888-394-3937
www.blindness.org

Glaucoma Foundation

116 John St., Suite 1605
New York, NY 10038
212-285-0080 or 800-452-8266
www.glaucoma-foundation.org

Glaucoma Research Foundation

200 Pine St., Suite 200
San Francisco, CA 94104-2713
415-986-3162 or 800-826-6693
www.glaucoma.org

Lighthouse International

111 E. 59th St.
New York, NY 10022-1202
212-821-9200 or 800-829-0500
www.lighthouse.org

Low Vision Council

111 E. 59th St., 12th Floor
New York, NY 10022-1202
www.lowvisioncouncil.org

Macular Degeneration Foundation

P.O. Box 9752
San Jose, CA 95157
408-996-7989 or 888-633-3937
www.eyesight.org

National Alliance for Eye and Vision Research

426 C St., N.E.
Washington, DC, 20002
202-544-1880
www. eyeresearch.org

National Association for Visually Handicapped
22 W. 21st St.
New York, NY 10010
212-889-3141
www.navh.org

National Eye Institute
National Institutes of Health
2020 Vision Place
Bethesda, MD 20892-3655
301-496-5248
www.nei.nih.gov

National Federation of the Blind
1800 Johnson St.
Baltimore, MD 21230
410-659-9314
www.nfb.org

National Library Service for the Blind
and Physically Handicapped
Library of Congress
1291 Taylor St. N.W.
Washington, DC 20011
202-707-5100
www.loc.gov/nls

Prevent Blindness America
500 Remington Road, Suite 200
Schaumburg, IL 60173-4557
847-843-2020 or 800-331-2020
www.preventblindness.org

Resources for Rehabilitation
33 Bedford St., Suite 19A
Lexington, MA 02420
781-862-6455
www.rfr.org

Glossary

accommodation. An adjustment of the lens to change its focusing power and sharpen the definition of objects you're looking at.

acuity. How sharply or clearly you can see something at a distance. Someone with normal visual acuity is said to have 20/20 vision, which means that he or she can see objects clearly from 20 feet away that most people with normal sight are able to see clearly from 20 feet away.

anterior chamber. The space between the iris and the cornea. This area is filled with a fluid called aqueous humor.

aqueous humor. A clear fluid that fills the anterior chamber. It nourishes the cornea and the lens and helps maintain the internal pressure of the eye.

astigmatism. A focusing problem that occurs when your cornea is not curved evenly in all directions. Typically what you see is distorted more in one direction than in others.

atrophy. The shrinking, thinning or wasting away of a tissue or an organ, such as that which happens to your retinal pigment epithelium if you have macular degeneration.

blepharitis. An inflammation along the edge of the eyelids that can cause irritation and itching.

capillary. Any of the tiny blood vessels that form networks throughout the body, such as in the retina.

cataract. A clouding of the normally clear lens of the eye that causes your vision to blur.

chalazion. A relatively painless swelling on the eyelid caused by blockage of a small oil gland within the eyelid.

choroid. A thin layer of arteries and veins sandwiched between the retina and the sclera. The choroid plays an important role in nourishing the retina.

cones. Light-sensitive cells of the retina that provide your central vision and allow you to see fine detail and color.

conjunctiva. A thin, moist, clear membrane that covers the exposed front portion of the sclera and lines the inside of your eyelids.

conjunctivitis. An inflammation of the conjunctiva that gives your eye a reddish or pinkish coloration.

cornea. A domed layer of clear tissue at the front of the eye. The cornea works with the lens to focus light entering the eye.

dermatochalasis. An age-related drooping of the eyelid skin. This condition may cause the upper eyelid to sag over your eyelashes and interfere with your vision.

diabetic retinopathy. A complication of diabetes that damages the tiny blood vessels that nourish the retina. Diabetic retinopathy is brought on by high blood sugar levels. If untreated it can lead to blindness.

dilation. The action of enlarging or expanding, such as the change in pupil size that occurs when you dim the lights or use dilating eyedrops.

drusen. Clumps of waste deposit that form under the retinal pigment epithelium. They appear as yellow dots behind the retina in the back of the eye. Drusen signal the beginning of macular degeneration.

ectropion. A condition that develops when the tissues of the eyelid relax, causing the eyelid to sag and turn outward from the eye.

edema. Swelling of tissue due to the presence of an abnormal amount of fluid. Macular edema may cause vision problems in more severe forms of nonproliferative diabetic retinopathy.

entropion. A condition that develops when the eyelid turns in toward the eye.

farsightedness. A focusing problem in which you can see objects that are far away clearly, but objects that are near to you appear blurry. The condition is also called hyperopia.

floater. A small bit of debris floating in the vitreous that can look like a spot, a hair or a string before your eye. What you're seeing is the shadow that this material casts on your retina.

fovea. A small depression in the center of the macula that contains only cone cells and provides your sharpest vision.

glaucoma. A group of eye conditions resulting in abnormally high pressure inside the eyeball. This pressure causes extensive damage to the optic nerve and loss of peripheral vision.

hyperopia. *See* farsightedness.

intraocular pressure (IOP). Pressure inside the eyeball that is maintained by the aqueous humor. An elevated IOP can signal glaucoma.

iris. The colored part of your eye. The iris contains a ring of muscle fibers that can expand or contract the size of the pupil.

lacrimal glands. Tear-producing glands located under the brow bone, just above your eyes.

lens. A clear, elliptical structure located behind the iris and the pupil. It works with the cornea to focus light entering the eye. The ability of the lens to thin or thicken allows it to change its focusing power. *See* accommodation.

low vision. Any eye problem that can't be corrected by standard eyeglasses, contact lenses or surgery. It's often the result of eye diseases such as macular degeneration, glaucoma or diabetic retinopathy.

macula. A dark reddish patch at the center of your retina that is densely packed with cone cells. The macula is essential to your central vision and allows you to see fine detail.

macular degeneration. A condition that occurs when tissue in the macula, the part of your retina responsible for central vision, deteriorates. The condition is also known as age-related macular degeneration (AMD).

myopia. *See* nearsightedness.

nearsightedness. A focusing problem in which you see objects that are near to you clearly, but objects that are farther away appear blurry. The condition is also called myopia.

neovascularization. The abnormal formation and growth of blood vessels, such as that which occurs under the retina when you have wet macular degeneration, and in the vitreous when you have proliferative diabetic retinopathy.

optic disk. The location where the optic nerve forms at the back of the eyeball. It's visible on the retina as a yellowish circle.

optic nerve. A bundle of nerve fibers that carries the visual information gathered by your retina to the visual cortex of your brain.

orbit. A socket that protects and cradles your eyeball. It's formed by a structure of heavy bone that includes the cheekbone, the forehead bone, the temple bone and the bridge of your nose.

point of focus. The location within the eyeball where visual information is most sharply focused by the cornea and the lens. The best sight occurs when the point of focus is directly on the retina.

presbyopia. A focusing problem that occurs when your lens loses its elasticity and ability to thicken or thin. It makes it difficult to focus on objects close to you.

ptosis. A condition that develops from a weakening of the muscle that raises your upper eyelid. This may cause the eyelid to droop over your eye and partially block vision.

pupil. The dark spot in the center of your iris — in reality a hole — through which light passes into your eye.

refraction. The bending of light waves by the cornea and the lens as light passes into the eyeball. Refraction allows images to be sharply focused and clear.

retina. A thin layer of tissue on the inside back wall of your eyeball containing millions of light-sensitive cells and other nerve cells that receive and organize visual information. The retina is connected to the brain by the optic nerve.

retinal detachment. A condition that occurs when the retina separates and pulls away from the choroid. If untreated this condition almost always leads to blindness.

retinal pigment epithelium (RPE). A layer of tissue forming the outermost surface of the retina. Deterioration of the RPE plays an important role in macular degeneration.

rods. Light-sensitive cells of the retina that provide your peripheral vision and allow you to see in dim light.

Schlemm's canal. An open channel behind the trabecular mesh-work that allows aqueous humor to drain from the eye.

sclera. A tough, white, leathery coating that forms the circular eyeball shape and protects the internal structures of the eye. It's also known as the white of your eye.

sty. A painful, red lump, resembling a boil or a pimple, on the edge of your eyelid. It's caused by a bacterial infection.

trabecular meshwork. A sievelike system of spongy tissue through which aqueous humor passes before draining from the eye through Schlemm's canal.

20/20 vision. A measure of visual acuity that means you can see objects clearly from 20 feet away that most people with normal vision are able to see from 20 feet away. To get a driver's license, you usually need at least 20/40 vision in one eye (with corrective lenses). That means a road sign you see clearly from 20 feet away can be seen clearly by a normal-sighted person from 40 feet away. Legal blindness is often defined as 20/200 vision (or worse) in your better eye, even with a corrective lens.

visual acuity. *See* acuity.

visual field. The area in front of you that you can see at a given moment without moving your eyes. It's made up of both your central vision and peripheral vision.

vitreous. A clear, gelatinous substance that fills the vitreous cavity. It helps maintain the shape of the eyeball and its internal pressure. It's also referred to as vitreous humor.

vitreous cavity. A chamber inside the eyeball extending from the back of the lens to the retina. It's filled with vitreous.

Index

Note: Glossary definitions are indicated by the **boldfaced** page numbers.

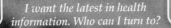
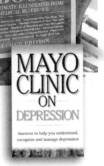

Now have Mayo Clinic health information at your fingertips day and night!

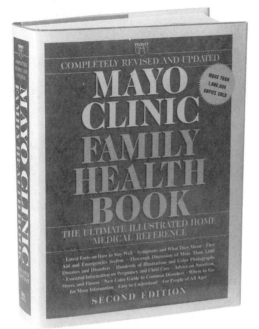

Mayo Clinic Family Health Book is a comprehensive resource that draws on the expertise and experience of more than 400 Mayo physicians, scientists, nurses, health educators and other health-care professionals.

A complete family health encyclopedia in one amazing volume –

- Color atlas of the human anatomy
- Guide to the 8 stages of life: from newborn babies to the elderly
- Best ways to stay well through nutrition and lifestyle
- Illustrated guide to first aid and emergency care
- Prevention and treatment of more than 1,000 ailments
- Photographic guide to common skin disorders
- How to get the most out of today's health care system
- Dictionary of common medications
- The diagnosis and treatment of cancer in children and adults
- Guide to medial tests

You'd have to purchase dozens of other health books to get all the information contained in this one volume!

Get answers with these best selling books from Mayo Clinic!

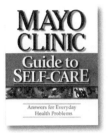

Mayo Clinic Guide to Self-Care
Product # 270100 • ISBN # 0-9627865-7-8
$19.95

Take the anxiety out of common health problems with this useful how-to book. *Mayo Clinic Guide to Self-Care* explains what you can do for yourself and when to seek medical attention. It describes how to respond effectively to medical emergencies. This book also covers what you can do to prevent or manage specific conditions, such as arthritis and asthma. You'll find that *Mayo Clinic Guide to Self-Care* provides hundreds of solutions to everyday health problems.

The Mayo Clinic | Williams-Sonoma Cookbook
Product # 268300 • ISBN # 0-7370-0008-2
$29.95

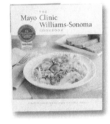

Eating well has never been easier — or tastier. Mayo Clinic has joined forces with the nation's leading cookware retailer, Williams-Sonoma, to offer the ultimate guide to preparing healthy and delicious meals every day. Winner of the 1999 Julia Child Cookbook Award and the World Cookbook Award, *The Mayo Clinic | Williams-Sonoma Cookbook* features a delightful collection of healthy appetizers, side dishes, entrees and desserts. Accompanying each of the 135 recipes is a full-color photograph, a complete nutritional analysis, useful cooking hints and nutrition tips.

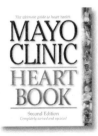

Mayo Clinic Heart Book, Second Edition
Product # 268150 • ISBN # 0-688-17642-9
$29.95

Whether you want to keep your heart healthy or you have some form of heart disease, you'll find *Mayo Clinic Heart Book*, Second Edition, is the ideal personal reference. Completely revised and updated with 100 illustrations and 75 full-color images, this book makes it easy to understand the normal functions of your heart. It also walks you through the most effective strategies for managing and preventing heart disease — including use of medications and recommendations for a heart-healthy diet and lifestyle.

Available at your favorite bookstore, or you may order direct by calling 1-877-647-6397. Order code 251.

(Price does not include shipping, handling or applicable sales tax.)

This series of books from Mayo Clinic has answers you're looking for!

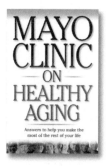

Mayo Clinic on Healthy Aging
Product # 270400 • ISBN # 1-893005-07-0
$14.95

Heredity and genetics play active roles in the aging process. Making better health and well-being decisions today can delay or even alter the effects of aging. This book offers guidance on how to make appropriate lifestyle choices that could lead to living a happier, healthier and more secure life.

Mayo Clinic on Managing Diabetes
Product # 270300 • ISBN 1-893005-06-2
$14.95

Diabetes can negatively affect health in many ways, including increased risk of blindness, kidney failure, heart disease and lower extremity amputations. This book includes discussions on the underlying causes of diabetes and offers insight on how to monitor, manage and live with diabetes.

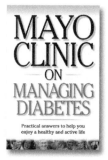

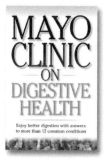

Mayo Clinic on Digestive Health
Product # 268900 • ISBN # 1-893005-04-6
$14.95

Digestive problems are common, but they shouldn't be ignored. This easy-to-understand book focuses on a variety of digestive symptoms, including heartburn, abdominal pain, constipation and diarrhea. It's a comprehensive guide to understanding why digestive problems occur, what you can do to manage or prevent them, and when you should see a doctor.

Other Mayo Clinic books include:	Product #	Price
Mayo Clinic on Chronic Pain	268700	**$14.95**
Mayo Clinic on High Blood Pressure	268400	**$14.95**
Mayo Clinic on Prostate Health	268800	**$14.95**
Mayo Clinic on Healthy Weight	270200	**$14.95**
Mayo Clinic on Arthritis	268500	**$14.95**
Mayo Clinic on Depression	270500	**$14.95**

Available at your favorite bookstore, or you may order direct by calling 1-877-647-6397. Order code 251.
(Price does not include shipping, handling or applicable sales tax.)

Keep informed ... with these award-winning monthly publications from Mayo Clinic

The Newsletter Devoted to the Health Concerns of Women

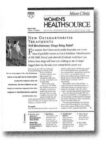

Mayo Clinic Women's HealthSource
Order code 9BK2
$27/year (U.S.)
$34/year (Canada)
$42/year (all other countries)

Your worst enemy as you get older isn't your own body. It's the body of misinformation and missed information that is standing between you and your peak health and vitality.

Now you can have access to the knowledge of Mayo Clinic health specialists through a newsletter devoted exclusively to your health concerns as a woman.

Each monthly issue is filled with reliable, timely news on women's health issues, including treatments, medications, health tips, testing and preventive care.

Get your health news from a source you know and trust, Mayo Clinic.

Features:

- Monthly columns on health tips, Headline Watch, Disease Dictionary and a readers question and answer section
- 12 issues a year
- 8 pages in each issue
- Monthly "Office Visit" article features an interview with a prominent Mayo physician
- Full-color medical illustrations
- 3-year index of articles

America's Most Popular Health Letter

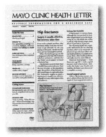

Mayo Clinic Health Letter
Order code 9BK1
$27/year (U.S.)
$34/year (Canada)
$42/year (all other countries)

Mayo Clinic believes that you can work with your doctor to improve your health in many ways, provided you have the latest and most reliable information.

That's the idea behind *Mayo Clinic Health Letter*, to put the world's most trustworthy health information in your hands each and every month.

From everyday health matters to serious diseases, every issue brings you practical information you can use!

Join more than 750,000 satisfied subscribers who read *Mayo Clinic Health Letter* each month.

Features:

- Monthly columns on Health Tips, what's in the news and a readers question and answer section
- 12 issues a year
- 8 pages in each issue
- 3 bonus medical essays a year, each focusing in-depth on a vital health issue
- Full-color medical illustrations
- 3-year index of articles

Order newsletters today by calling 800-333-9037.

MayoClinic.com

The health Web site from Mayo Clinic to visit ... again and again

It's innovative, new and available to you and your family at no cost! Take a few minutes to click through a trustworthy online resource from the health specialists at Mayo Clinic. Log on to MayoClinic.com where you'll find comprehensive coverage of more than 250 diseases and conditions, timely information about healthy lifestyles and disease management, personalized and interactive programs to help you improve your lifestyle, plus many more features all designed to help you take charge of your health. Join the millions of Americans who now use the Web to find health information that can make a difference in their lives.

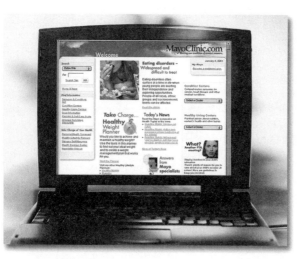

MayoClinic.com is your reliable source of health information on the Web.

Mayo Clinic Health Information
200 First St. S.W.
Rochester, MN 55905